Contents

Acknowledgements

This manual was prepared jointly by the Office of the United Nations High Commissioner for Refugees and the World Health Organization. Thanks are due to the following people who contributed to individual units of this manual:

Nick Argyll, Northwick Park Hospital, Harrow, Middlesex, England (Unit 2)

Nancy Baron, Family Rehabilitation Centre, Colombo, Sri Lanka (Unit 1)

Joop T.V.M. de Jong, International Institute for Psychosocial and Socio-ecological Research, Maastricht, and The Free University, Amsterdam, Netherlands (Units 2, 3 and 8)

Linda Gask, Research and Development for Psychiatry, University of Sheffield, England (Unit 3)

J.P. Hiegel, Medical Director, Oeuvres Hospitalières Françaises de l'Ordre de Malte, Phanat Nikhom, Thailand (Unit 6)

Richard Mollica, Director, Harvard Program in Refugee Trauma, Harvard School of Public Health, Boston, MA, USA, and Clinical Director, Indochinese Psychiatry Clinic, St Elizabeth's Hospital, Brighton, MA, USA (Unit 4)

D.S. Samarsinghe, Department of Psychiatry, Faculty of Medicine, Colombo, Sri Lanka (Unit 7)

Helmut Sell, Regional Adviser, Health and Behaviour, WHO Regional Office for South-East Asia, New Delhi, India (Unit 3)

Sima Wali, Executive Director, Refugee Women in Development Inc., Washington, DC, USA (Unit 9)

J. Williamson, Consultant, Refugee Children's Programmes, Richmond, VA, USA (Unit 5)

Many people gave valuable advice, including M.A.C. Dowling, Jim Lasselle and Marcus Wasserman. Sima Wali particularly acknowledges the use she made of the work of Neil Boothby and Elizabeth Jareg in preparing Unit 9. The draft version of this manual was reviewed by people working with refugees in many countries. The authors thank them all for their helpful comments.

The project which led to the production of this manual was coordinated by Giovanni de Girolamo and John Orley of the Division of Mental Health, WHO, Geneva, Switzerland.

The manual was edited by Joop T.V.M. de Jong and Lucy Clarke.

Illustrations are by Mary Jane Orley.

Introduction

Disasters and wars are happening constantly. One sure result is that some people have to leave their homes and countries and become refugees. While many refugees suffer physically from injury or hunger, far more suffer psychological harm. It is estimated that there are 18 million refugees in the world today, and twice that number of persons are displaced within their own countries. In the past, concern has often focused on the deaths, physical diseases and traumas that resulted from wars and disasters but nowadays there is also growing concern about the psychosocial and mental health consequences. Such consequences are not always short-lived; some can last a lifetime and some may even have an influence on the children of those affected. Yet in the midst of these negative experiences there may also be positive signs. Refugees should not be seen as helpless people who totally depend on help they are given. Refugees are often people with strong determination to survive, which is why they became refugees. People who provide help to refugees or other displaced persons should look for the capacity to survive and cope and try to help build up this positive element. In this way refugees and other displaced persons will be encouraged to use their own abilities to help themselves.

What can be learned from this manual?

This manual is intended to help those who work with refugees or other displaced persons to:

— recognize people with high levels of stress and teach them how to cope with their stress;

— understand what "functional complaints" are and recognize and help people with such complaints;

— help refugee women who have been raped;

— understand the mental health and development needs of refugee children;

— understand traditional medicine and work with traditional healers;

— recognize common mental disorders;

— deal with alcohol and other drug problems;

— help victims of torture and other violence.

Who is this manual for?

This manual is written primarily for relief workers, community workers, primary health care workers, primary school teachers and others who provide support to refugees and other displaced persons who have fled war or disaster. These personnel may be working for international organizations such as UNHCR, WHO, the United Nations Children's Fund (UNICEF), the Red Cross or Red Crescent Societies or other nongovernmental organizations (NGOs) active in this field. The whole of the manual will be relevant to many workers while others, according to their responsibilities, will find parts of it useful. It is written in simple language and the reader does not need special training in psychology or mental health. Health professionals may also find it useful, particularly as an aid for training and supervising others. The term "refugees", as used in this manual, should be understood as including all displaced persons.

Adaptation of the text

The manual provides broad guidelines, which should be adapted as necessary to the local culture. It may also be useful to translate the manual into the local language, even if the persons using it know English as a second language. The process of translation will help to put the principles set out in the manual into a form that is relevant to those who will use it, thus helping them to be more effective.

The need for tolerance and acceptance

Relief workers may or may not be of the same religion, culture or social class as the refugees themselves. If they are not, they should be encouraged to be tolerant of other religions, customs and beliefs. In difficult times, people need the support provided by their religions and customs, and relief workers should be aware of this. Refugees have left the security of their homes and they need to feel accepted in their new surroundings.

The mental health of the helpers

Finally, those who work with refugees and other displaced persons need to take care of their own mental health and put the principles in this manual into practice for themselves. A helper who is mentally exhausted cannot help anyone. Refugee workers need leisure time and the opportunity for healthy enjoyment of their life away from their work. The first unit of this manual aims to help workers prepare themselves for their role and help others as effectively as possible.

Useful helping skills

Learning objectives

After studying this unit you should be able to:

1. Understand yourself better.

2. Organize a treatment plan.

3. Create a safe helping environment.

4. Build a helping relationship based on trust.

5. Listen effectively and skilfully probe for information.

6. Provide appropriate comfort and support.

7. Encourage self-sufficiency.

8. Assess the needs of the person you are trying to help.

9. Develop a plan of action for the person you are trying to help.

To provide support and treatment to refugees with emotional difficulties a helper must learn some basic helping skills. This unit teaches the basic skills necessary to communicate effectively.

Becoming an effective helper

To be an effective helper you must first understand yourself better.

Why have you chosen to be a helper?

Ask yourself these questions:

- Why do I want to help others?

- What do I get from helping others?

- How might my personal needs or interests interfere with my ability to help others?

- What strengths do I have that will be useful in helping others?

People who choose to help others are providing a valuable service. Helping can be rewarding but it can also be difficult and stressful for the helper.

People have different reasons for choosing certain types of work. It is important to know yourself well and to understand your reasons for wanting to help. No one helps solely in order to do good for someone else. Often people choose to help others because it makes them feel worth while. Sometimes people have suffered themselves and want to be kind to others to repay kindness that was shown to them.

Some helpers may themselves have needed help in the past and remember what it was like to have no one to assist them. Others may at times have problems of their own and believe that, if they help others, they will also be helped to cope themselves. You must understand your reasons for wanting to help so you can be sure that they do not prevent you from helping others.

It is very important for helpers to have their own lives under control. It can be difficult to sense another person's feelings if your own problems fill your mind.

Who am I?

Explore your personality. Be clear about your values and beliefs.

The following is a list of personal attributes and goals. Try to understand which are most important to you. Number them in order from 1 to 18, with number 1 as the most important and number 18 as the least important. There is no single correct order. Each person has his or her own priorities.

health	friendship	world peace
basic life needs	inner strength	spirituality
self-respect	excitement	mature love
success	family security	wisdom
natural beauty	material wealth	adventure
minimal stress	satisfying sex	education

Ask friends or family members to number the items on the list according to what they feel is most important. Compare your lists.

Then ask a young person or elderly person to number the list. Compare the lists again. What did you find?

It is quite normal that people's values should differ. Each person is unique and each has a special way of experiencing the world.

For most refugees basic life needs and family security would be at the top of the list. It is difficult to concentrate on other values until these needs are met.

4

Personal characteristics of an effective helper

To be an effective helping person it is necessary to have the following personality characteristics:

genuine caring	calm manner	sense of humour
clear thinking	dependability	honesty
common sense	nonjudgemental attitude	self-confidence
self-awareness	positive attitude to life	respect for others
warmth	flexibility	openness.

Helpers must fully respect the persons they are trying to help, regardless of values and beliefs. You must recognize the differences between you and the person you are helping, and you must respect these differences.

You are not the judge of the other person's life; rather, you should think of yourself as an invited guest. You have been asked to help, not to take over people's lives.

Helpers should try to empathize with the persons they wish to help. This means trying as best you can to imagine yourself in that person's position and trying to understand how that person sees the world. Ask yourself: How does this person feel about his or her life? How does this person view the world? What is best for this person to do?

Do not assume that you know the way another person feels because that is how you would feel. Each person has a unique life history and a particular set of values, needs, desires and beliefs.

Nine steps to develop a treatment plan

These basic steps will help you develop a treatment plan for those you try to help.

1. Arrange a safe, quiet and private helping environment.

2. Build a helping relationship based on trust.

3. Listen effectively.

4. Probe for information.

5. Provide comfort and support.

6. Encourage self-sufficiency.

7. Assess the problems.

8. Develop a plan of action with the person you want to help.

9. Provide follow-up.

1. Arrange a safe, quiet and private helping environment

Refugees often have to live in cramped quarters without privacy. They have no choice but to adjust to this.

They may not feel that to talk with you is in their best interest. They may be afraid that everyone else will hear about their problems. If they do speak openly, they may run the risk of being talked about by others or of making others resentful or hostile. Knowing that others are listening, they may limit what they say so the helper cannot be sure of the real problem. Being a refugee often takes away a person's self-respect. Whenever possible the helper must help refugees to regain their dignity.

You can usually find a quiet place somewhere to talk. Go for a walk, sit in an empty school or doctor's room, or even go to the washrooms at meal-time when no one is there. Ask the refugee to help you find a place to talk. This will help to build trust and appreciation of your efforts.

2. Build a helping relationship based on trust

You must earn a person's trust through your behaviour. Helpers are not automatically trusted just because they are called helpers. Initially people will speak about their problems only in a superficial way. Over time, as you build trust, they will talk to you more fully. Only then will you really be able to help them.

Approach people gently. Most refugees have good reason not to trust others. Remember to try to put yourself in their position and understand how they feel.

3. Listen effectively

People often begin to feel better simply because they are given the opportunity to talk and believe they are being listened to. Trying to suppress feelings and not speak about them can be the cause of emotional and even physical discomfort. Trying to ignore, avoid or deny emotional sadness or pain causes a great deal of stress. Problems of depression, constant worry, uncontrollable fear, aches and pains that have no physical cause, and many other symptoms can result from feelings being held in and not expressed.

The helper's most useful role may often be to encourage the expression of feelings; to do this you must be a good listener.

How to listen

- Sit facing the person.
- Make eye contact.

- Give your full attention.

- Do not let yourself be distracted.

- Nod your head or say something like "I see", so the person knows you are listening.

Listening has many levels:

- We can listen to a person's words.

- We can listen to the sound of a person's voice.

- We can listen by observing how a person's body moves as he or she speaks.

- We can listen to silence and note what the person does not say.

- We can listen to the meaning the words have for the person who is speaking.

- We can listen for a person's feelings.

Never assume that you know how a person feels. Listen to what the person has to say.

Example

An elderly woman comes to a health clinic complaining about a headache. She wants medicine. If the helper listens only to her words, he will give her a pain-killer and send her home.

Helper's thoughts: I see her hands are trembling. I wonder if this is because of the head pain or something else. I will ask her for more details.

Helper: Please tell me more about the pain. Where does it hurt? Are there times when it gets worse?

Woman: It hurts on the left side of my head. A sharp pain. It gets worse with loud voices.

Helper: When did it begin?

Woman: Last week.

Helper: Tell me about the first time you noticed it.

Woman: I have always been healthy. Other old people have developed medical problems in the camp. Not me. I am strong. I always helped my daughter and her four children. But last week I suddenly had this pain. I stayed in bed.

Helper: Tell me about your life in the last week. Has anything been different?

Woman: Yes. My son-in-law returned after three years in prison.

Helper's thoughts: Her voice sounds sad and anxious. I did not hear the excitement or pleasure you might think she would feel.

7

Helper: What is it like to have him back?

Woman: Oh — it's nice.

Helper's thoughts: Again, no real positive feeling. It may only be a coincidence but her headache seems to have begun when her son-in-law returned. This is my guess. I need to ask more about her feelings.

Helper: How will your life change now that he is back?

Woman: My daughter will have to change her ways. We've done everything for the children on our own. We managed to eat and live without his help. He knows nothing about living in the camp. He doesn't know the children. The little one cries when he comes close to her. Everyone in the camp knows he was in a political prison.

Helper's thoughts: Now I know why she has a headache. The pain-killer would not cure this headache. Her son-in-law's return has a meaning I could never have guessed.

4. Probe for information

You need to have a great deal of information to be able to understand a person's real problems. You get this information by asking questions and probing for details.

Information-seeking skills

Probing

Ask questions calmly and slowly. Don't insist. Avoid sounding like an interrogator.

Be thoughtful about what you ask. Think about how the person may feel in answering you.

Let people talk at their own pace.

Questioning

Questions that are closed and require only a yes or no answer (such as "Are you afraid?") provide little information. An open statement that probes for information is more useful — for instance, "Please tell me about what is frightening you."

Leading

Lead the conversation to get information, but continue to follow the person's train of thought. If the person is talking about lack of food, don't immediately ask about the children's schooling. If you want to know about the children, direct the conversation from lack of food to the children's diet and health and then on to their schooling.

Types of information

Everyone has behaviour, thoughts and feelings. To help someone with an emotional problem it is necessary to understand how behaviour, thoughts and feelings contribute to the problem. Probing, questioning and leading can be used to get information about all three areas.

Behaviour

Many people ask for help by talking about a problem of behaviour: "I have a headache", "My heart races", "My child refuses to go to school", "My husband and I argue", "I don't have enough money", "I cry all the time", "I can't think clearly", "I don't want to have sex."

It is easiest for the person to begin by describing behaviour. To understand fully the behaviour, ask for details that enable you to envisage what the person's daily life is like and ask the person to describe the problem exactly.

People may make their problems worse by their own behaviour. You may, for instance, find that people behave in ways that are self-defeating.

Thoughts

Ask what the person thinks about the problem. What really are the thoughts going on inside the person's mind?

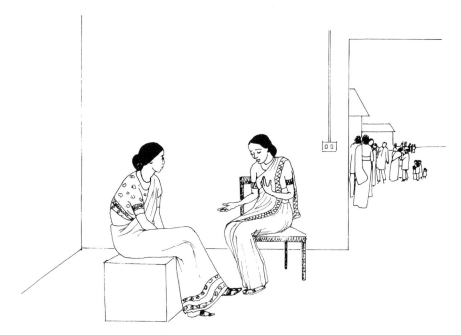

Try to find out a person's inner thoughts

9

Many people constantly talk to themselves in negative terms. They say: "I can't do it", "I am a failure", "I am no good", "I am stupid."

Example

A young widow comes to talk to you and complains, "I cry all the time."

Helper first asks about the behaviour: Tell me about when you began to cry so frequently.

Widow: After my husband died I cried, but then it stopped. Recently I tried to train for a job and I didn't get the job. Then I began to cry all the time.

Helper: What are you thinking when you cry?

Widow: I think that my life is terrible and it can never be better.

Helper: Do you think there is anything you can do to make your life better?

Widow: I think that I am too stupid. There is nothing I can do.

From this you learn that this person's inner thoughts have led her to convince herself that she is incapable.

Feelings

It is very important to try to understand people's feelings. People should be encouraged to express feelings openly. This is often difficult because many cultures discourage expression of feelings in this way and people believe they must always appear confident and strong.

If you provide a safe environment, appear caring and listen closely, most people will eventually open up about their feelings. Once they realize that expressing feelings is permitted, the feelings often come out like a flood. Encourage the flow but be careful not to overdo it. People who seem to be saying too much should be slowed down, but be careful not to silence them completely.

People will tell you their feelings and may often show them as well. They may cry or get angry or show frustration or stress. This is good and should be encouraged. Holding those feelings inside can cause emotional and physical problems.

It can be stressful for the helper to listen to a person expressing emotions in this way. Stay calm and resist the impulse to try to make the person feel better at once. First, the feelings must be expressed. This is not the time to make a plan for improvement or to give advice; it is the time to listen and probe for information. It is no use being too logical; feelings are not usually based on logic.

If the person begins by describing behaviour, start there with your probing. Next move on to finding out what the person thinks and eventually find out about feelings.

Example

Young man: I can't sleep at night. I need pills.

First the helper examines the young man's behaviour.

Helper: How long have you had difficulty sleeping?

Young man: One month.

Helper: Is it difficult every night?

Young man: Most nights.

Helper: What is different on the nights you can sleep?

Young man: I keep the lights on all over the house.

The helper tries to understand the person's feelings.

Helper: Tell me what you feel when you lie in bed.

Young man: I feel tired.

You can see from the response that the helper asked about feelings too soon. The person was not yet ready to share his feelings. So the helper asks about thoughts.

Helper: What thoughts do you have as you lie in bed?

Young man: I think about when the soldiers came and took me into detention.

The young man becomes tearful. The helper makes a comforting statement.

Helper: Those must be painful thoughts to have night after night.

Young man: Yes.

More tears. The helper wants to encourage the young man to express his feelings. The helper does not want to make him feel better yet, but wants him to feel that someone empathizes with his pain.

Helper: I know it can be difficult to share such painful feelings. Take your time. When you are ready, please tell me more about what you feel.

Young man: I lie in bed and listen for every sound. The quiet is scary. Little noises are scary. I start to sweat.

More tears.

Helper: What frightens you the most?

Young man: I think the soldiers will come again and this time they will kill all of us.

5. Provide comfort and support

There are many ways to let people know that you hear not only their words but also their emotions. Your genuine emotional response is the most powerful way. If you feel tearful, don't try to hide it. Many of the feelings and stories of refugees are very sad.

How to provide comfort and support

- Use a kind and gentle voice.
- Your body can show your interest and caring. Sit close, but not too close, and lean towards the person.
- Offer a tissue for the person's eyes or a drink of water.
- Show concern in your facial expression.
- If appropriate, touch the person's arm to show concern.
- Respond to how the person feels, not to how you feel. If a man tearfully tells you the story of his forced move to the refugee camp, listen and comment, "I can hear how sad it was for you."
- Take care that your show of concern does not make the person feel uncomfortable and stop the flow of emotions.
- Many times a person will feel tremendous relief after speaking openly and knowing that someone listened and cared.

6. Encourage self-sufficiency

Helpers should encourage the self-sufficiency of those they want to help. Although you are available to help at a difficult time, your usefulness is temporary.

You should show that you have confidence in their capacity for self-help. Many people feel uncomfortable if they are in need of help. If you behave in a way that implies you think you know what is best, you can make people feel even more incompetent.

Feeling dependent or helpless can make people angry and resentful and this makes problems worse. Most refugees had normal lives before they had to move. You should express respect for the fact that the person has survived a terrible experience and belief that, although this is a difficult time, the person possesses the strength for self-help. Help people to find their strength again. If you do things for people, or tell them what to do and how to do it, you are communicating a message that you feel they are incompetent. Help people to help themselves. There is an old proverb:

If I give you fish you eat for a day.
If I teach you to fish you eat for a lifetime.

12

7. Assess the problems

Before you can develop a plan of action you need to assess the problems. Spend some time thinking about what the person has told you. Often the problems presented to you initially are not the only issues to be considered.

- Consider the person's behaviour, thoughts and feelings and how each contributes to the problem.

- Consider the person's life situation and the practical difficulties to be faced in making the change that is needed. Some ways of tackling the problem may not be available to the person because of poverty, restriction of movement or physical risk due to political conflict or other reasons.

- Consider the person's family and community. What impact do other people have on the person you are trying to help?

After considering all this information, try to make a first assessment of just what the problems are that need to be addressed.

People's feelings about their problems may change after their conversation with you. When you next see them, ask how they now view their problems. What do they now think are the problems that need to be dealt with?

Be flexible with your ideas. Both you and the person you are trying to help need to have a similar understanding of the problems so that you can work together to develop a plan of action.

8. Develop a plan of action for the person you want to help

State the problems clearly

The assessment should have helped you both to define the problems clearly. State the problems that need to be worked on.

Determine the goals

Clarify the goals that the person is trying to reach. For example, the person you are trying to help may state the problem as: "I am always tired." Ask what the person's goal is. The person then may respond, "I want to have enough energy to cook dinner for my children."

Decide which problem to tackle first

If there are many problems, put them in order of priority and work on one at a time.

Set up the plan of action

You and the person you are trying to help should discuss possible ways of working on the problems. There are many ways to reach a goal. As you help people, offer them ideas and encourage them to come up with others. People should choose the course of action that is best for them.

Discuss how it will feel to succeed. People are often afraid to feel good or to succeed in achieving their goals. Examine both the benefits and the problems that success will bring. Ask how the person's family and community will feel if he or she succeeds. Other people can have a tremendous influence. The person may be worried that success may have both positive and negative effects.

Try to find out what people will do if their plan fails. How will they feel? How will they boost their confidence to try again? What will they do next?

You may be tempted to give specific advice and tell people what to do, especially if a person specifically asks, "What do you think I should do?" Be careful. People do not really want to be told what to do. Often they are stuck in negative patterns and need help to see alternatives. A person needs to be able to choose how to proceed. This will also encourage self-confidence.

Written record

It is often useful to write down the plan of action. Some people benefit from having a copy of a written plan. Here is one way of writing a plan of action.

Plan of action

Name: . . . .   Date: 2 August 1995

Follow-up: Meeting with helper in one month to check progress.

Problems	Goals	Improvement plan
1. Daily headaches	To reduce the number of headaches	Do relaxation exercises every morning
2. Loneliness and isolation	Make one friend	Each morning spend at least 15 minutes with a neighbour
3. Daughter behaves aggressively towards other children	Improve daughter's behaviour	Watch daughter at play with other children. Show her other ways to behave when she becomes upset. Enrol her in preschool.

The person takes action

The person now uses the plan of action as a basis for working towards self-improvement.

9. Provide follow-up

The type of follow-up will vary from case to case. In some situations you will need to meet the person regularly. Setting up a schedule of meetings is part of the plan of action. People need to know that you are dependable and that you will see them regularly. In other cases you will see the person only occasionally, possibly only once. Try to set up a plan of action that the person feels confident in doing independently.

Sometimes it is better to have fewer goals so that the person is more likely to be successful. The feeling of success often helps a person to be more ambitious the next time goals are set.

When people recover it is important that they feel that their own efforts gave them success. This way they will feel confident to help themselves in future. If they praise your efforts and not their own, their self-confidence will not improve. Your most important goal is to help people to help themselves.

UNIT 2

Stress and relaxation

Learning objectives

After studying this unit you should be able to:

1. Understand how people find themselves under high levels of stress.

2. Identify people under high levels of stress.

3. Advise people how to deal with their stress.

4. Use group activities to help deal with stress.

5. Tell people about stress.

6. Teach relaxation exercises.

7. Understand how massage reduces tension.

8. Advise people how to sleep better.

9. Teach breathing exercises.

All refugees experience stress. Some suffer more than others from its effects. Many causes of stress can be prevented or reduced, thus greatly improving a person's mental and physical health.

Why people find themselves under high levels of stress

Some stress is normal. When people feel threatened, they have a natural and positive tendency to defend and protect themselves or to flee. These reactions can be seen by an increase in muscle tension, quicker breathing and a faster heartbeat. When people feel that the threat is over, they relax. During this relaxation their muscles grow soft, their heartbeat slows down and they breathe more slowly and regularly. They feel calm and are able to rest and restore their energy. In most people these reactions of activation and relaxation are in balance.

Refugees, however, often experience enormous amounts of stress. This may be because they do not know where their relatives are, or because they feel insecure about their future, or for various other reasons. Refugees may continue to be distressed even when there is no direct threat. Because of this, their muscles may feel tense all the time. This tension can cause physical complaints which may in turn worry them. These worries may then increase the tension in their muscles and make the physical complaints worse. In other words, they get caught in a spiral of increasing anxiety and physical complaints.

Relaxation exercises can help to break this spiral of tension and physical complaints. By learning how to reduce tension, people feel more relaxed and can rest better. They worry less at moments when they do not need to worry and their physical problems trouble them less.

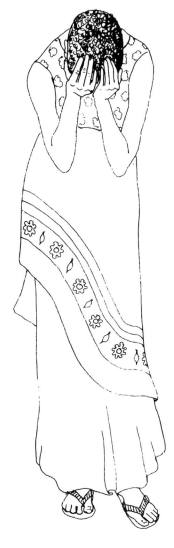

Individuals under stress can suffer from tiredness, headaches and other problems

How to recognize people with high levels of stress

Stress comes from unpleasant experiences and living conditions. It can disturb the mind and body. Stress causes unhappiness and prevents people from doing useful work. It is important to identify people who are suffering from a lot of stress.

A person's behaviour may also create or reduce stress. Following simple advice and using relaxation techniques can give relief from stress.

Stress may affect all areas of a person's life, causing:

— mental distress;

— physical symptoms;

— changed behaviour;

— problems in relationships with other people.

Individuals suffering from stress often do not complain about stress directly. Instead they complain of many different physical and mental symptoms. They may even develop illnesses that require medical treatment.

Symptoms and signs of stress

Individuals under stress may have any of a variety of symptoms.

Symptoms of stress in the mind

- Anxiety or getting angry easily.
- Sadness, crying or feelings of helplessness.
- Moods that change quickly.
- Poor concentration, needing to be told things several times before understanding and remembering them.
- Thinking about the same things again and again.

People may find it hard to describe their symptoms.

Symptoms of stress in the body

- Tiredness.
- Headache.
- Tense muscles.
- Palpitations or irregular heartbeat.

- Feeling as though one cannot get enough air.

- Nausea (feeling sick) or pains in the abdomen.

- Poor appetite.

- Vague pains, for example in the arms, legs, or chest.

- Disturbed monthly cycle in women.

Fatigue or intense tiredness

One of the problems many refugees experience is a very strong fatigue or intense tiredness. Tiredness can be caused by many physical complaints such as anaemia. If you feel that people you are trying to help have any physical complaints, refer them to a doctor.

Tiredness can, obviously, also be caused by lack of sleep. Find out whether the person you are trying to help has somewhere comfortable and quiet to sleep. For more advice on helping people to sleep better, see page 28.

Also remember that fatigue or intense tiredness can, in itself, be a symptom of stress. All the techniques in this unit can help people who have fatigue caused by stress.

People may have many different symptoms which come and go. If someone has a fever or is losing weight or develops symptoms that do not go away, advise him or her to go to a health centre. For example, chronic stress may cause an ulcer. The health worker can check for other causes of stomach pains such as inflammation of the stomach which may be caused by hookworm or excessive use of alcohol, sometimes together with malnutrition.

Symptoms of stress in behaviour

- Reduced activity, no energy.

- Overactivity and inability to rest (restlessness).

- Taking alcohol or drugs such as cannabis or opium to relieve tension.

- Difficulty in concentrating on one task.

- Sleep problems (reduced or disturbed sleep, too much sleep or sleep during the day).

Someone who cannot do useful work, for no obvious reason, may be suffering from stress. To be sure that the person does not have a more serious disturbance such as depression or panic attacks, see Unit 4, *Common mental disorders*.

Symptoms of stress in relationships with other people

- Lack of emotion.

- Arguments and disagreements.

- Too much dependence on others for decisions and support.

How to find out the cause of the person's problems

It is important to talk to members of the family or to others who know the person well. First you need to know if the current behaviour is normal for this person. Then you should ask in what ways the individual's state is not normal.

Try to find out about the possible causes and nature of the stress. Ask carefully about the experiences people have gone through. Find out about their current position and the future plans of the family or community. What is their political and legal status? Will they have to move again? Is there any information available about missing relatives or friends?

It is important to realize that the symptoms and signs listed above can sometimes be found in people with chronic functional complaints (also called somatizers), people suffering from depression, people suffering from anxiety disorders, or people who drink too much alcohol.

If a person has a *functional complaint*, the physical symptoms are the expression of an underlying personal or social problem. It would be useful to study Unit 3, *Functional complaints*, before you start to try to help these people.

People with *depression* have more serious complaints. They are more irritable and sad, have no energy and lose weight. Depressed people not only have difficulty falling asleep but they also wake up early. Often they do not do things that are normal in their culture, like chatting with people, taking part in rituals or preparing meals. They may have had the problem before; their depression may have come and gone in the past. The ways in which depression differs from stress are dealt with more fully in Unit 4, page 42.

People with *anxiety disorder* also have more serious complaints. They may have symptoms like sweating, hot and cold flushes, a pounding heart, and strong feelings of anxiety or panic. The difference between stress and anxiety disorder is dealt with in Unit 3. During panic attacks, people may breathe in an unusual way. This is called hyperventilation. The treatment for hyperventilation is dealt with on page 29.

You can often recognize people who are *drinking too much alcohol* by the smell of alcohol or the trembling of their hands (see Unit 7, page 101).

If the family or person has gone through very shocking experiences, first read Unit 8, *Helping victims of torture and other violence*, page 110. If you decide that the person needs counselling, as described in Unit 8, first do the relaxation exercises as described in this unit. Do not start the counselling as in Unit 8 until you have taught the relaxation exercises described in this unit.

Advising people how to deal with stress

People need to be encouraged to change their behaviour in order to:

— restore the normal pattern of sleep at night, and engage in useful and enjoyable activity in the day;

— find positive ways of dealing with stress;

— stop harmful ways of dealing with stress.

People under stress find it difficult to relax and should be taught special relaxation exercises. These are the most important aspect of treating someone with stress. There are many ways of relaxing, such as reading, singing, listening to music or just resting. Ask people what they normally do to relax and encourage them to go on doing it.

Try to put isolated individuals or families in touch with others from the same area or at least of the same culture and language. Even in a crowded camp, people can be very lonely.

People who feel helpless should be encouraged to do some useful activity, however limited. They should also talk to stronger or more optimistic people in the community, especially religious leaders.

Crowding and other restrictions cannot always be avoided, but make sure that individuals under stress take advantage of whatever facilities are available. Check that they are getting food, water and medical care for illness.

Rest at night is essential. Encourage the community to reduce noise at night. If necessary, establish quiet hours, such as between 22:00 and 06:00.

People who are looking after children and others who need care may feel over-burdened. Try to find others in the family or community who can help. Even an hour or two of relief from caring for children can be a great help.

Advise people to stop using alcohol or drugs. Even too much coffee or black tea can be harmful and prevent proper relaxation.

Physical strength and personality are hard to change. Under stress, weaknesses become more obvious. When stress is removed and people get enough rest their strengths will return. Under stress some people become anxious or unhappy; some cause unhappiness in others too. Conflict between people can be due to stress. When this happens, rest, relaxation, and separation of those arguing may be the best solution. If serious problems exist in a relationship, ask older or more stable people to help resolve them. Encourage people not to waste energy on arguing but to use their energy productively together to solve the problems that they all face.

Dealing with stress through group activities in the family or in the community

Stress can affect whole groups of people. Stress in an individual causes physical and mental distress. Stress in a community leads to arguments, low morale, low productivity and crime.

Normal communities have social activities that help reduce stress. These include music, dancing, singing, celebrations and sports. They allow people to meet together and be happy together. It is very healthy to enjoy oneself. Even with poor living conditions and plenty of reasons for sadness, such social events should be encouraged. No one should be lost in sadness all the time.

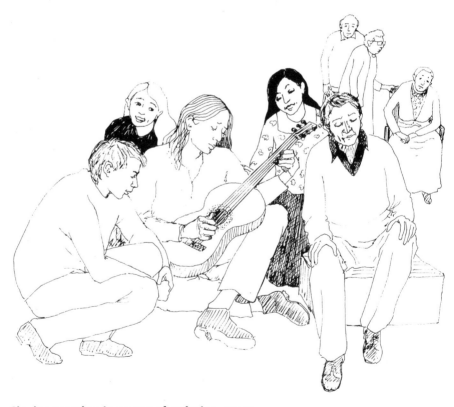

Singing together is a way of reducing stress

Refugees often feel isolated because they have left some of their family behind. Meeting other people with whom they can enjoy activities and share worries is an important way of reducing stress. It helps people cope with this difficult phase of their life.

Celebrations need not be elaborate. Music, singing and dancing require little or no equipment or money. Celebrating special cultural and religious days helps people who have had to leave their country. Celebrating birthdays is a way of celebrating life and hope for the future.

Sports and games not only provide physical exercise, but also bring people together. Children usually play spontaneously but adults may need encouragement. Find people in the community who will take responsibility for organizing sports and celebrations.

Doing useful work makes up a large part of normal daily life. It is often not possible in refugee camps or similar settings. The usual domestic tasks of cooking, washing and looking after children are still there but there may be no possibility for work outside the home. Remember that refugees who may seem helpless were once living productive lives and may be used to hard work. Productive activity is good therapy. Try to stimulate productive activities. If necessary, ask the refugees to form a group to make administrators aware of the need for collective or productive activity. People who are enabled to work feel less helpless and useless. Working in groups allows the strong to encourage the weaker ones.

Educating people about stress

People under stress can be supported both within a group or as individuals. The first step in this supportive process is to inform and educate them about stress.

People under stress need to be educated to recognize and deal with their stress. Many of the causes of stress are obvious to anyone yet people often do not realize that stress is causing their symptoms. Proper understanding of stress reassures people that they do not have a physical illness and are not going crazy. They also need to know that they can help themselves recover.

People can learn to help themselves and get help from others. Just as sleep relieves tiredness, stress is relieved by simple relaxation exercises that anyone can learn.

It is normal to be tired after a day's work and sleep usually relieves this tiredness. But sleep is not always enough, so we are not always totally fresh and happy when we wake up. In this way, stress builds up from day to day. It stops the mind and body from working properly. Different problems arise in different people, depending on which part of them is weakest. When the body and mind get enough rest they will heal themselves.

Alcohol and drugs must not be used to combat stress. Their pleasant effects last only a short time. Their harmful effects last longer. They can make stress worse and do great damage to mind and body. Alcohol and drugs will make anxiety, depression and sleeping problems worse and will reduce appetite and strength. They can also lead to loss of family, friends and the ability to work.

Stress affects the whole community. No one should feel that only he or she has this problem. When recovering from stress everyone needs help from other people.

As a refugee worker you can identify people under stress. You can educate them about stress and teach them relaxation exercises. You should also educate their family and friends about the needs of a person under stress. Relatives and friends can give practical help by making sure that the stressed person gets proper food and drink and keeps to a regular routine of rest and activity. They can also look after children and give love and emotional support. The family should encourage positive activities and not concentrate on the individual's physical and mental complaints. It is important to avoid criticism and conflict.

Sometimes individuals become very distressed, perhaps because of very severe stress such as that caused by the absence or death of relatives. Other people can be supportive just by being with them and quietly listening to or comforting them.

If there are many people who have been separated from their families and are now by themselves, bring them together in pairs or small groups. Ask them to take responsibility for each other and take care of each other.

Even when conditions are very bleak everyone should have some useful activity. This makes people feel more able to improve their situation.

Text to read or hand out to people under stress

I want to tell you something about stress and how you can help yourself by learning relaxation exercises.

Our body and our muscles are much more active than we think. When people are anxious or brooding they often squeeze or tense their muscles. This is why we use expressions like "tense expectation" (use an expression from your own culture, if possible). Is this bad? Yes and no. Often it is not bad and may even be very positive. Being afraid is a kind of alarm so it is very useful. It alerts people and prepares them for quick action. Therefore your body and your muscles become tense when you are afraid. You have to be ready to act, to run, to fight or to jump. For example, maybe you heard that an enemy was approaching the place where you lived. Maybe you got scared, your body became tense and you escaped.

Unfortunately people also often worry about things they do not need to worry about. Sometimes people continue to worry when the threatening situation is over or is not really dangerous any longer. Some people worry about minor problems. For example, people try to do their best in their life but they always wonder whether what they do is good enough. This creates unnecessary fear and worries which in turn may lead to tension in the body. In the long term this can be harmful. When muscles stay tense for a long time this can lead to physical complaints such as pain in different parts of the body.

This creates an additional worry. Someone who is stressed does not feel well and may live in difficult circumstances. The person may get less pleasure from playing with children, from talking to people, or from making love. In other words, fears and worries lead to muscle tension which can result in bodily complaints. These complaints increase the fears and worries, which lead to more muscle tension and so on. People may feel as if they are in a spiral of constantly increasing anxiety.

If a person succeeds in reducing tension, physical complaints will be reduced and will be easier to handle. The person will feel more relaxed and will be better able to cope with worries. People will have more energy to deal with the real problems they face.

To become really relaxed you need to exercise daily. Like a child learning to walk or to talk, you need to practise relaxation. Gradually you will learn to relax. You will get more control over the tense feelings, and be troubled less by the complaints.

Try to find a quiet moment and a quiet place. You can do the exercises with your partner or with other family members who feel stressed. Make sure that you are not disturbed by other people.

Teaching relaxation exercises

Exercise first with a colleague or a friend. Ask the other person to comment whether the pitch, rhythm and speed of your voice help them to relax. Pause for 4–6 seconds between phrases. Pause for about 10 seconds when you change the exercise from one part of the body to another. The relaxation exercise below should take about 15 minutes.

During the first two weeks try to do the exercise at least twice a week with the whole group or the individual you want to help. If you have a tape recorder, record the exercise, give the tape to the participants, and ask them to exercise daily. From the third to the fifth week ask the participants to exercise twice a day for 10–15 minutes. They can do this on their own. Forgetting part of the text is no problem; just doing the exercise will be enough. After about six weeks the participants can exercise in situations and at times when they find it difficult to cope.

Text for relaxation exercise

You are lying on the floor. Your eyes are open and you are looking at the ceiling. Close your eyes.

Feel yourself lying on the floor. Feel how heavy you are. Press the heel of your right foot hard against the floor. Feel the muscles in your right leg becoming hard and stiff. Now release the pressure of your heel against the ground and sigh. Feel your right leg becoming soft and relaxed. Lift your right leg a little way above the ground. Feel the muscles you need for this. Your left leg is doing nothing and is lying motionless on the floor. Lower your right leg back to the floor. Feel your right leg lying heavily on the ground. Your right leg is feeling tired. You can feel the warmth in the muscles of your right leg.

Press the heel of your left foot hard against the floor. Feel the muscles in your left leg becoming hard and stiff. Now release the pressure of your heel against the ground and sigh. Feel your left leg becoming soft and relaxed. Lift your left leg a little way above the ground. Feel the muscles you need for this. Your right leg is doing nothing and is lying motionless on the floor. Lower your left leg back to the floor. Feel your left leg lying heavily on the ground. Your left leg is feeling tired. You can feel the warmth in the muscles of your left leg.

Now press the muscles in your buttocks together. You can feel the lower half of your body becoming hard and stiff. Now stop squeezing and sigh. Feel the lower part of your body becoming soft and relaxed. Feel your pelvis lying broadly and heavily on the floor.

Press your right hand hard against the floor. Feel the muscles in your right arm becoming hard and stiff. Now release the pressure of your right hand against the ground and sigh. Feel your right arm becoming soft and relaxed. Lift your right arm a little way above the ground. Feel the muscles you need for this. Your left arm is doing nothing and is lying motionless on the floor. Lower your right arm back to the floor. Feel your right arm lying heavily on the ground. Your right arm is feeling tired. You can feel the warmth in the muscles of your right arm.

Press your left hand hard against the floor. Feel the muscles in your left arm becoming hard and stiff. Now release the pressure of your left hand against the ground and sigh. Feel your left arm becoming soft and relaxed. Lift your left arm a little way above the ground. Feel the muscles you need for this. Your right arm is doing nothing and is lying motionless on the floor. Lower your left arm back to the floor. Feel your left arm lying heavily on the ground. Your left arm is feeling tired. You can feel the warmth in the muscles of your left arm.

Press your shoulders hard against the floor. Feel the muscles in your shoulders becoming hard and stiff. Now release the pressure of your shoulders on the ground and sigh. Feel your shoulders becoming soft and relaxed. Feel how warm and heavy your shoulders are.

Press your head hard against the floor. Feel the muscles in your neck becoming hard and stiff. Now release the pressure of your head against the ground and sigh. Feel your neck becoming soft and relaxed again. Now lift your head a little way above the floor. Feel the muscles you need for this. The rest of your body is doing nothing. Now lower your head to the ground. Feel how heavy and tired your head is. Put your hands on your stomach. Feel your stomach becoming warm. Put your arms alongside your body again. Feel your whole body. The warmth, the weight, the relaxation.

Another type of relaxation exercise

This is another, more mental, relaxation exercise. It may fit more easily in your culture or in the culture where you are working. It is an easy and pleasant exercise.

- Sit comfortably, preferably in a quiet place, with your feet flat on the floor.
- Close your eyes.
- Breathe easily through the nose.
- Fix your attention on your muscles and feel how they become a little more relaxed every time you breathe out. Do this for two to three minutes.
- Now imagine that each time you breathe in you take in energy and health. Every time you breathe out you get rid of some tension and stress. Do this for two to three minutes.
- Now remember some pleasant and beautiful place you have visited in the past. Imagine you are there now. Let your mind rest easily in this place.
- When other thoughts come into your mind, just watch them come in and go out again. You see that thoughts come and go by themselves. Even worrying or unpleasant thoughts will go if you do not pursue them.
- You are resting deeply in a pleasant place. Remember what it looks like, sounds like, feels like. Let other thoughts come and go on the surface of your mind.
- After about 10 minutes say goodbye to this pleasant place, but remember that you will return there again.
- Take some deep breaths and then open your eyes.

This exercise can be done as often as you like, at least once a day.

Physical exercise

Physical exercise is necessary for good health and is useful in reducing stress. Even someone who is very tired — after a long journey, for instance — should have some exercise each day. Walking is very good exercise, especially for those over 45 years of age or in poor health. Younger people should do something more active — swimming, football or whatever is suitable in the circumstances.

(If daily life in the camp already requires a lot of walking then many people will not need this advice.)

Simple massage

Massage is widely used in many cultures to relieve tension and promote health. Find out what is common in the culture of the refugees and whether there is anyone who can help teach and give massage.

People can massage themselves, or other members of their family; parents can massage their children. The ideal time for massage is in the morning as part of the daily washing or bathing routine. If vegetable oil is available, it should be used. Oil is best if slightly warmed.

If there is time, massage the whole body. Use the whole hand to massage firmly up and down the long bones of the arms and legs. After travel, massage of the soles of the feet is particularly soothing.

As well as reducing tension, massage promotes health.

Ways of improving sleep

Proper sleep is very important both for avoiding stress and for coping with it. Getting proper sleep is part of staying healthy. The body's rhythm of waking and sleeping should be in tune with the rhythm of day and night.

People with stress often have trouble falling asleep, or they wake up in the night. They may sleep during the day. Explain the importance of a regular routine. Everyone should have a regular bedtime.

Remind people that, even if they are not asleep, resting quietly in bed is good for them. Most people who think that they lie awake the whole night usually sleep quite a lot without knowing it. Ask the family or neighbours of a person under stress to help keep things quiet at night and to go to bed at about the same time every night. A regular routine is very important.

People should, however, associate their bed with the idea of sleep. Therefore a person who has not gone off to sleep after half an hour should get up for a while and wait until feeling sleepy again, and then go back to bed. If the person is still awake after another half an hour, he or she should get up and repeat the procedure.

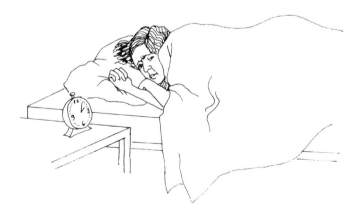

People with stress often have trouble falling asleep

Rules that will help restore normal sleep

- Do not smoke, eat or drink during the night.

- Do not read or listen to music at night and avoid listening to the radio or watching television late into the evening.

- Avoid coffee and black tea, especially in the evening.

- Eat your evening meal no later than 19:00 if possible.

- Do not take alcohol or drugs. They may put you to sleep but they destroy the normal pattern of sleep and you will wake up feeling bad. Avoid sedative medicines and never take them without a doctor's advice.

- A warm sweet drink (e.g. milk, but not coffee or tea) is good before bedtime.

- A light walk in the evening also helps, but not heavy or energetic exercise.

- Avoid arguments in the evenings.

- Do not sleep during the day, unless a short rest in the afternoon is normal for the climate and culture.

- The area between the eyebrows may be massaged gently and slowly for a few minutes before sleep.

Breathing exercises

Before starting breathing exercises with anyone, explain what hyperventilation is and what to do about it.

Hyperventilation

What is hyperventilation?

Some people complain of not being able to get enough air, even though there is nothing wrong with their lungs or heart. They feel anxious or faint and may have tingling sensations in their hands or lips. They may have a tight feeling in their chest. They may feel dizzy. (But remember, dizziness can also be caused by anaemia or low blood pressure.) Others see mist before their eyes, or their heart may pound. People have these complaints because they are breathing too much or breathing incorrectly. The harder they try to breathe, the worse they feel. Some people start breathing wrongly by taking deep breaths. It is better not to breathe too deeply.

What to do

Two simple things can help:

- Breathe slowly and deeply (but not *too* deeply). Pause slightly between breaths.

- Breathe with the abdomen and diaphragm, not with the chest and ribs. To teach people this, do the exercise below.

Text for breathing exercise to stop hyperventilation

Lie on the floor or on a bed. Put both hands on your stomach between your navel and your groin. Feel your abdomen with your hands. You can feel the warmth on your hands. Breathe in so that your stomach swells up and becomes round. Breathe out so that your stomach goes in again. Breathe in so that your stomach swells up and becomes round, breathe out so that your stomach goes in again.

Concentrate on the movement of your stomach for a while. Feel how relaxed and heavy you are becoming. Your thoughts are fading away. You are starting to feel good.

When you have done these exercises you will feel heavy, warm and comfortable. Your breathing is calm. I will now count to five:

One, start to move your feet and legs.

Two, start to move your hands and arms.

Three, move your head.

Four, open your eyes, look at the ceiling.

Five, stretch completely from your toes to the tips of your fingers.

The breathing exercise below will take about 5 minutes. First, try it with a colleague or a friend.

Text for a breathing exercise

Lie on the floor or on a bed. Place your hands on your stomach. Close your eyes or turn them towards your stomach. Feel the parts of your body that are in contact with the floor or the bed — your heels, your calves, your bottom, your back, the back of your arms, and the back of your head. Try to relax your stomach so that your breathing can reach the lower part of your stomach in a natural way. Pay close attention to the movements of your stomach and your hands.

Count to two slowly in your mind while breathing in. Then count to four when breathing out. Wait patiently until you feel the natural need to breathe in again. Breathe quietly the way you usually do.

I will now start counting with you. 1, 2; 1, 2, 3, 4, and a pause; 1, 2; 1, 2, 3, 4, and a pause; 1, 2; 1, 2, 3, 4, and a pause; 1, 2; 1, 2, 3, 4, and a pause; 1, 2; 1, 2, 3, 4, and a pause.

Go on like this until you feel you are breathing steadily.

(The "1, 2" to breathe in should take about 3–4 seconds, the "1, 2, 3, 4, and a pause" to breathe out, about 10 seconds.)

The person can practise this exercise as often as he or she likes. It should help the person to breathe normally at all times.

Other ways to cope with stress

Many cultures have a way of meditating. Find out whether there is anyone in your community who can teach meditation. Experienced teachers would be a great help. The ways of meditating used in the culture can be as effective as the other methods of reducing stress that have been described in this unit. They may in fact be more effective because people are familiar with them.

Most meditation techniques require:

— a quiet atmosphere;

— a comfortable posture;

— a "mental device" (a word, a sound, a symbol);

— a passive mental state.

This is true not only for relaxation techniques but also for yoga (e.g. hatha-yoga), elements of Sufism, Buddhism and Taoism, reciting verses from the Koran and certain forms of mysticism.

UNIT 3
Functional complaints

Learning objectives

After studying this unit you should be able to:

1. Recognize people with functional complaints.

2. Understand that serious psychological or psychiatric disorders may be causing functional complaints.

3. Help people who have functional complaints.

Every health worker (and relief worker) knows people who tell a long story about many vague physical complaints. Although the health worker asks many questions to find out if these complaints relate to a specific disease, it is still not clear what disease the person is suffering from. Sometimes the health worker is almost sure what disease is producing these complaints, but then the person has other complaints that do not fit into the normal pattern of the disease.

The health worker may also feel that these people with vague and varied complaints are different from others. Sometimes they seem to insist too much about their complaints. They seem to worry more than is necessary about their unidentifiable illness. The health worker may find it difficult to interrupt such people as they talk about their complaints. Some of them will not give clear answers to the health worker's questions.

Often such people have been to many health workers and local healers without finding relief. They may have used a variety of medicines without feeling any better. Others have had their stools, their urine or their blood examined several times. Even when a parasite or a disease was found and treated, their complaints continued or went away only for a short time.

When people behave in this way the health worker may feel irritated, uneasy or even powerless. Sometimes the health worker will prescribe some medicine and hope that the person will not return. However, a couple of weeks later, the person comes back with the same or similar complaints. This can all be very frustrating.

What are functional complaints?

Persons such as those described above have the following features:

- They have physical complaints, but it is hard or impossible to detect a disease.

- They may have many symptoms or vague symptoms, such as "pains all over the body" or "feeling weak all the time".

- They may have a minor disease, but this disease cannot account for the numerous or vague physical problems that they complain of.

These complaints are called "functional complaints" or "somatizations". People with this problem are sometimes called "somatizers", "chronic (neurotic) complainers" or "functional complainers". The term "functional complaint" is used because the complaint seems to have a function or use for the person.

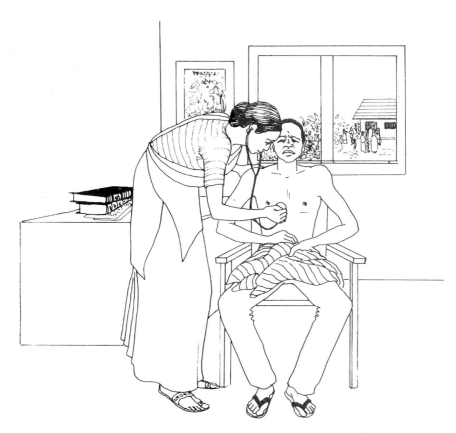

People with functional complaints may have been to many health workers without finding relief

People with functional complaints are very common in any situation where health care is provided. Some 20–30% of adults who come to a health care facility have this kind of problem. In stressful situations this problem can occur even more often. When a refugee camp is threatened from outside, or when people are afraid about their legal status, complaints such as these often become more common.

What function do these complaints fulfil?

- Some people have an underlying personal or social problem. They find it hard to talk about this problem but find it easier to talk about physical complaints. Some are afraid that if they talk about their personal problems, they may be thought of as mentally ill.

- Some people may think that this is the way to talk to health workers or relief workers. They may have been taught that you go to a health facility to talk about physical complaints. Taking the role of someone who is ill may be easier than explaining a personal problem.

- Their culture may have taught them to express their problems through their body. It is as if the culture prescribes that, when you have personal problems, you may express them through the body.

- Some people may not realize that they have personal problems. Yet the stress created by these problems shows itself in their bodies. This is explained in Unit 2, *Stress and relaxation*.

- Some people feel that certain sensations or feelings in their body are painful or threatening. Everyone feels pain now and then but some people pay more attention to these sensations.

- The last possibility is that these complaints are symptoms of a more serious disorder. The complaints might be a symptom of depression, anxiety disorder or alcohol abuse, or they may be the consequence of serious violence, torture, or rape (see Units 8 and 9).

How to recognize underlying serious psychological or psychiatric disorders

Depression

As described in Unit 2, people with depression usually have serious complaints: they are irritable and sad, have no energy and lose weight. Most depressed people have difficulty falling asleep. Often they also wake up too early. In the morning they may again be troubled by feelings of sadness or by their functional complaints.

Depressed people may feel unable to do things that are normal in their culture, such as chatting with people, attending ceremonies or preparing a meal. They may feel hopeless or have difficulty in seeing any worthwhile future. They may lose interest in life, and suffer from lack of energy and constant tiredness.

Depressed people may have had a similar problem before; their depression may have come and gone several times.

For more about the difference between someone with functional complaints and a depressed person, see Unit 4, page 42.

Anxiety disorder

Like the complaints of persons suffering from depression, anxiety disorders are more serious than functional complaints. People with an anxiety disorder may have symptoms such as sweating and hot and cold flushes. The heart may pound, and the person may suffer from strong feelings of anxiety, panic or worry. Ask questions such as "Do you ever feel really panicky and tense?" Unit 4 explains more about the difference between functional complaints and anxiety disorder.

The panic attacks may be accompanied by incorrect breathing, which is called hyperventilation. The symptoms and the treatment of hyperventilation can be found in Unit 2, page 29.

Alcohol abuse

You can often recognize people who are drinking too much alcohol by the smell of alcohol or the trembling of their hands. For more information, see Unit 7, page 101.

Violence or torture

Some symptoms may be a consequence of serious violence or torture. This may be the case when people complain that they:

— think all the time about a painful experience from the past;

— feel as though they are undergoing the same experience again;

— have bad dreams and nightmares;

— have lost interest in life;

— have poor concentration, poor memory, or tell the same story over and over again;

— feel afraid or nervous.

35

If the person or the family has suffered extreme violence, see Unit 8, page 110.

How to help people with functional complaints

This section outlines nine steps to help people with functional complaints.

Step 1

Make sure the person is examined physically.

If you are a relief worker without medical training, refer the person to a health worker. Ask the health worker to give the person a medical check-up. Tell the health worker (personally or by letter) that you think that some personal or social problem may be behind the complaints. Ask the health worker to make a diagnosis and to provide treatment. Ask the health worker to send the person back to you if the complaints do not disappear or if there really do seem to be other problems behind the complaints.

If you are a health worker, examine and treat the person as described above. Avoid unnecessary examinations or referrals to specialists or laboratories unless you think the person has a serious physical disease.

Step 1 is important because if there is a physical disease you need to take care of it. You are also showing that you respect the person. By taking the complaints seriously you can build up trust. If there is no physical disease, you will need that feeling of trust for the following steps.

Step 2

Tell the person the results of the examination and the treatment.

Step 3

Reassure the person that the symptoms are not the beginning of a serious illness.

Recognize that there is a problem but tell the person that this problem will not lead to more serious illness. Say that you can tell that the symptoms are real, even when there is no clear physical cause.

Never say, "There is nothing wrong." For the person with the problem, something is certainly wrong.

36

Do not give medicines. Giving medication will make it more difficult for the person to understand what is causing the complaints. It will also stop you from working towards solving the underlying problem.

Step 4

Explain in simple words that people sometimes find the normal functions of their body painful or threatening.

It is wise to suggest this in general terms without referring to the person's own complaints. Explain that everyone at some time experiences pain. You might say, for example, "We all feel pain and discomfort. We all have headaches or cramps in our stomach now and then. This is part of normal life."

Step 5

Explain in simple words how bodily symptoms can be caused by emotional reactions or problems.

If the person does not believe you, you could say, "When people are anxious they get tension in their neck muscles and this causes headaches." Or you could mention a saying in the local language that explains the link between stress and complaints. (Every language has expressions like "Worrying too much makes your knees weak" or "Many sorrows turn your stomach into a stone".)

If the person finds it difficult to see the link between the complaints and the underlying social and personal problems, do not argue that such a link exists. This kind of psychological understanding is not necessary to help the person.

Instead, ask how the complaints affect the person's life. A woman may tell you she has less time to care for her children and that this makes her husband angry. The answer will often give you a hint of the underlying social or personal problem or tell you what is really causing the complaints.

Step 6

Help the person to relax (see Unit 2).

Step 7

Help the person to solve the social and personal problems.

Step 5, above, will help start this process.

Simply listening to the person may already be a help. Also talk about the person's problems and ask about or give advice on changes that could be made. An easy way to do this is as follows:

- Make a list of what the person regards as the problems, in order of importance.

- Sort out together which problems can be tackled given the circumstances in which the person lives.

- Help the person to think of different ways to solve the problems and select the best way to solve them one by one.

- Encourage the person to take action and see how it improves the situation.

- Talk about the positive aspects of the action.

Step 8

Try to find out if there are other resources available, such as family members or friends.

Can they provide any form of social support? Also find out if the person can be involved in productive activities that might help to generate income or to rebuild self-esteem.

Step 9

Be firm in not giving medicines, but also invite the person to visit you again.

The person should not think that your refusal to give medicines means that you want to break the contact. Suggest another visit in one or two months "to keep in touch and see how you are doing".

Common mental disorders

Learning objectives

After studying this unit you should be able to:

1. Understand how to identify and manage mental illness in refugees according to five general rules.

2. Interview a person effectively.

3. Describe the most common symptoms of:

   — depression;

   — psychotic episodes;

   — mental disorder due to long-term psychosis;

   — mental disorder caused by hurtful and frightening events;

   — mental disorder caused by beatings or other injuries to the head;

   — emotional disturbances associated with intense fear and worry;

   — emotional disturbances related to poor sleep.

4. Identify and manage patients who are suicidal, "confused" or "out of control".

5. List the names and appropriate doses of some medical drugs used in the treatment of each illness.

6. Understand the use of counselling, family support and community support as well as traditional and religious healing in managing people with mental disorders.

Five general rules for identifying and managing mental illness in refugees

To help you to identify and care for refugees from your community who are mentally ill, you should learn these five general rules. Use them to help you when you interview refugees.

Rule 1

Learn the names your culture uses for emotional distress and mental illness.

You may not be a religious or traditional healer, but you need to know how religious and traditional healers identify and treat emotional distress and mental illness. During the first meeting with patients ask them the names of the illnesses they believe they have. Ask their family members the same question. Ask what traditional medicines the patient has already received, if any. This information will help you understand what the community feels is wrong with the person. It will help you know if traditional healing has helped.

You might also be working with medical doctors and nurses. Learn your culture's names for mental illness and the ways of dealing with it. Then you will be able to share this information with the health workers. This will help them to understand the patient's illness better.

Rule 2

List the common symptoms of mental illness in your community.

Get to know the many different ways refugees may reveal that they have a mental illness. Keep this list ready so that you can compare it with the complaints of persons you deal with.

Rule 3

Always try to make a home visit.

A home visit enables you to observe a person's living conditions. Many of the problems will become obvious to you. Ask the husband or wife, family and friends if they believe the person has a real mental illness. Why do they believe this? They have been observing the person for a long time. They can tell you facts that the person has omitted, wants to deny or is too upset to tell you.

Rule 4

Use simple terms that are easy to understand when asking refugee patients about a possible mental illness.

For example, if you are trying to find out if a person is hallucinating, ask in simple words, "Are you hearing voices that other people cannot hear?"

Rule 5

In the first meeting with persons you want to help, tell them that you will not tell anyone anything they say or anything about them without their permission.

Everything a person tells you should be kept private. This will protect the person from employers, camp administrators, family members and others who may want to find out something that the person wants to keep private. If you tell anyone a person's history or secrets, the person will never trust you again.

Interviewing to identify the causes of mental illness

When you interview someone with a mental illness, you should try to identify the causes of their symptoms so that you can help them. The following suggestions should help you do this:

- Try to interview the person alone in a quiet place away from the noise of a crowded health centre. Remember, no one should overhear the person's conversation with you.

- After the first interview the person will know that you will keep what he or she says private. Now you can interview the person's family and friends, either with the patient or separately. Ask them to tell you what they think is wrong with the person. Ask what treatment the person has received. Has the treatment worked?

- Find out the folk diagnosis or name used by the community to describe the person's problems. Remember, what the family or community think is wrong with the person may not be correct.

- Before the interview prepare a list of questions to ask the person who is seeking your help. If you follow this list, you will not miss important information.

- Ask specific questions such as "Do you have nightmares?" Avoid general requests like "Tell me about your difficulties".

- If the person is able to answer you clearly in the first interview, ask whether he or she has experienced torture or other hurtful and terrifying events.

- Do not ask a woman if she has been raped, even if you suspect that she has. Once the woman trusts you, and believes you will keep the information secret, she will mention it.

- Find out exactly what the person expects of you. Always ask, "What do you think I can do to help you?"

- If you suspect a physical cause for the symptoms and you cannot identify it, refer the person to a doctor or nurse.

- Always try to offer some hope of relief from suffering — but never do this unless you mean it.

Depression

Many refugees suffer from depression. Mental illness due to depression can be very serious and may lead to suicide. The symptoms of depression may also be disabling and prevent the refugee from studying, working and enjoying any activity.

The most common causes of depression are loss of a family member or friend, and the sickness or death of a child. Other common causes are the loss of valuable property and extreme poverty. Another cause of depression may be a shameful or embarrassing event within the community such as an unwanted pregnancy, the break-up of a marriage or being fired from a job. Hurtful and terrifying experiences such as rape, or being attacked and robbed by bandits, can also cause depression.

In some depressed people, you will not be able to find a cause. Some depressions seem to happen for no identifiable reason.

Almost all refugees at times feel sad and hopeless about their situation. But even with these feelings, most do not suffer from the mental illness called depression. Depressed people feel very sad and hopeless for months. Nothing gives them pleasure. They believe that nothing and nobody can help them in their suffering. They do not seek help because they believe their situation cannot be improved.

Symptoms

The most common symptoms of depression are:

— overwhelming sadness and deep sorrow;

— hopelessness;

— thinking about harming oneself;

— crying easily;

— worrying constantly;

— anxiety, tension;

— lack of joy in life;

— lack of energy, easily becoming tired;

— physical complaints such as headaches that do not go away;

— poor sleep;

— weight loss;

— lack of interest in sex;

— difficulty in paying attention or remembering;

— feeling "bad", worthless or less respected than other people.

Depressed people often complain of physical symptoms. Take care not to be distracted from the main underlying psychological disorder.

How to identify people who are depressed

1. Find out in your first interview if the person is suicidal. Ask directly, "Do you think life is not worth living?"

   If so, ask, "Would you prefer to be dead?"

   If so, ask, "Have you thought of killing yourself?"

   If so, ask, "Have you tried to kill yourself or have you plans to kill yourself?"

   If so, ask, "Do you want to kill yourself?"

   Find out if the person has a plan. Also ask about previous suicide attempts. Ask when, how and how many times these attempts have been made.

2. Find out if the person has all the other symptoms of depression. How long have the symptoms lasted? Ask the person if the symptoms have interfered with his or her activities at home, school or work. Ask the family the same question.

3. Ask both the person and the family what event or events have occurred to cause the depression.

4. Some depressed people will deny feeling sad and hopeless. They will deny having problems even if something bad has just happened to them. These people will have many of the physical complaints that indicate emotional distress in your culture. Check your list and compare it with the person's complaints. The symptoms will have no medical cause and will not respond well either to modern medication or to traditional herbs and folk remedies. Ask, "How many doctors, nurses and folk healers have you visited?" "Have their treatments helped?" "Why not?" Find out from the wife, husband or other member of the family what personal or social events make the person's physical complaints worse.

5. Patients who are very depressed may hear, see or smell things that do not exist. Ask direct questions that test for this, such as "Do you sometimes hear voices when there is no one there?" If people hear voices, ask if the voices are ordering them to kill themselves or others. If they say "Yes", ask, "Do you feel you are able to resist these voices telling you to kill yourself?"

Some depressed people will also say they are having upsetting feelings, which may be associated with death. For example, they smell dead bodies or feel they are infested with snakes or worms. If a person has these feelings, ask the family if the person has any false beliefs such as that he or she has cancer. Is the person mistakenly convinced that he or she has a deadly disease?

How to help people who are depressed

1. First ask yourself: "Is this person suicidal and capable of self-harm?" Read the following list and check off all those statements that apply to the person you are trying to help. Depressed people to whom any of the statements apply are more likely to kill themselves.

   - The person hears, smells or sees things that do not exist. People who hear voices telling them to kill themselves or others are particularly dangerous.

   - The person falsely believes that he or she is going to die.

   - The person has a detailed plan for suicide or for killing family members.

   - The person has made attempts at suicide in the past.

   - The person suffers from a fatal illness.

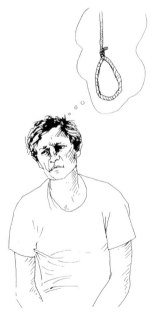

A person with a detailed plan for killing himself is more likely to commit suicide

- The person lives alone and cannot be supervised or protected from harm.

- The person drinks alcohol or uses drugs.

- The person has easy access to a means of killing himself or herself (e.g. poison, weapons or grenades).

2. Persons who are suicidal should be admitted to hospital immediately or kept under observation at home or in a community centre until they can be trusted not to hurt themselves.

3. If someone has just attempted suicide, try to judge how serious the person's depression is. Find out, by using the above list, whether the person is still suicidal. If people remain a danger to themselves, ask the doctor or nurse to keep them in hospital until it is safe to let them go home. Such people should probably be started on treatment with medical drugs. You may also begin counselling. If people in this condition leave hospital too soon, they may try to kill themselves again. Indeed, some will succeed in killing themselves.

4. Once a depressed person is safe from self-injury, you can join with the family and friends in trying to solve the social and personal problems that lie behind the depression. This help can begin in the hospital.

5. Ask traditional and religious healers to help the depressed person overcome his or her hopelessness, guilt or shame.

6. Do not blame or criticize people who are depressed. It will only make them feel worse. Allow them to solve their problems slowly with your help.

7. Encourage the person to return to work or school as soon as possible. Explain to both the person and the family that once the depression goes away, he or she will feel well again.

8. Depressions and suicide attempts associated with rape and sexual violence need special counselling skills. Refer these people to counsellors who know how to counsel rape victims. If this is not possible, follow the guidelines on rape in this handbook (see Unit 9).

If a medical doctor is available to examine and treat the person:

9. A doctor may prescribe drugs such as imipramine, amitriptyline or similar medicines, up to 75–150 mg at bedtime. It is best to start with 25 mg and work up to higher doses over a week or so. Watch out for side-effects such as a dry mouth, blurred vision, irregular heartbeat and lightheadedness or dizziness, especially when the person gets out of bed in the morning. Persons with heart disease should have a thorough examination before starting the medication.

10. People who are agitated (cannot stay still, walk around all the time), or who have strange beliefs or hear voices when no one is there, may be given a tranquillizer as well as one of the antidepressants mentioned above. The kind of tranquillizers used for this are chlorpromazine or haloperidol.

11. Remember that a person who seems depressed, but who does not improve with counselling and medication, may have a physical illness. It is particularly important that a person who is not getting better should be examined by a doctor.

Acute psychosis

A person may be brought to you who is "out of control" or "confused".

An "out of control" refugee has lost the ability to listen to anyone. People who are out of control may shout loudly and threaten to hurt themselves and others. Or they may sit quietly in a room and refuse to answer your questions or respond to your instructions.

A "confused" refugee will not be able to tell you where he or she is, or what time of day or day of the week it is. Confused people will not be able to tell you what they are doing or why. They may not even be able to tell you who they are. A confused person may become out of control.

How to identify people with acute psychosis

1. It is quite easy to identify people with acute psychosis. They will be brought to your attention by family, friends and members of the community who are worried about their strange behaviour or risk of violence to themselves and others. It would be typical, for example, for a person with acute psychosis to hide in a room with a blanket over the head. If you ask questions, you will be given answers that make no sense. People who are out of control will not respond to anything you say to try to calm them down.

2. Find out from the family if the behaviour of the person has changed suddenly. What event may have caused this change?

3. Remember, confusion and uncontrollable behaviour can be caused by many medical problems, such as:

   — acute infections such as malaria or other common diseases;

   — vitamin deficiency (e.g. pellagra);

   — withdrawal of alcohol or drugs;

   — head injury.

   A sudden emotional shock such as rape or the death of a child can sometimes also cause this condition.

46

4. The person's confusion may not be due to a medical problem but to a mental illness associated with chronic psychosis (see page 48). The acute psychotic episode may be the beginning of this illness.

How to help people with acute psychosis

1. Treat people with acute psychosis gently and calmly, and offer reassuring words of support.

2. Put them in a quiet room in a home or a clinic where there is not much noise. There should be nothing dangerous that they can grab to hurt themselves or others. The situation can be made worse by noise and too many people being around.

3. Restrain a refugee who is out of control. Do not do this in a rough way. Ask the family and friends to help you. Ask for help so that neither you nor the person you are restraining will get hurt. Never try to restrain someone by yourself.

4. Once the person is in a safe environment, ask a few people (usually family or friends) to supervise until there is no longer a risk of harm to anyone.

5. Ask the doctor or nurse at the health centre to examine the person as soon as possible. If a person's confusion has a medical cause this should be treated properly by a doctor or nurse. This usually takes place in hospital.

If a medical doctor is available to examine and treat the person:

6. Try to arrange for drugs to be given to calm a person who is dangerous and out of control. The doctor may have to give a tranquillizer such as haloperidol or chlorpromazine to get the person safely to a health centre or hospital.

   - For the most uncontrollable people the health centre or hospital staff can give haloperidol. They can give 5 mg into the muscles every hour, up to a total dose of 15 mg.

   - For less disturbed people, it may be enough to give 1–2 mg of haloperidol by mouth 2–5 times a day. If necessary, they may be given 2 mg of haloperidol into the muscles every 4–6 to hours up to a total dose of 15 mg. When the person has become less disturbed, haloperidol medication can be given in a single dose at night.

   - Side-effects of haloperidol may include stiff muscles, restlessness (not being able to sit still), drooling saliva and rolling the eyes to the back of the head. To prevent these side-effects, trihexyphenidyl should be given orally in doses of 2 mg once or twice a day.

   If haloperidol is not available, chlorpromazine can be used. The most disturbed people will probably need 25–50 mg of chlorpromazine given into the muscles. The dose may be repeated after one hour if the person has not calmed down and it can be given every hour until the patient is quiet, up to a total dose of 200 mg.

- Chlorpromazine injections can be changed to oral medication as soon as the patient is cooperative enough to take the drug by mouth because the injections can be very painful.

- Less disturbed people can be given 100 mg of chlorpromazine twice or three times a day by mouth as tablets or syrup. Watch out for dizziness and lightheadedness when using this drug.

- If the person complains of side-effects similar to those described above for haloperidol, trihexyphenidyl should be given.

7. A person whose condition has a medical cause will need to be treated by staff in the health centre. Any mental disorder should be treated in addition to the medical problem.

8. If the person's condition is caused by a mental illness, such as chronic psychosis, this condition must be treated (see next section).

The difference between acute and chronic psychosis

Some people are psychotic (unfortunately people often call them "crazy" or "mad") for a short while. This "acute psychosis" can last for days or weeks. It may occur once or several times in a person's life.

Some other people are psychotic for longer periods. They may seem quite well and behave quite normally some of the time, but at other times they behave in strange ways which do not fit the "normal" behaviour of their community. At the beginning of a period like this, they may seem to have an acute psychosis but this is a long-term problem that needs long-term treatment. These people suffer from "chronic psychosis".

Chronic or long-term psychosis

In any refugee community there may be people with chronic psychosis. When they first come to your attention, they may seem to have acute psychosis. If left untreated, these people can have many more acute psychotic episodes. Over time, their family life, work or school performance may suffer because of their illness. You need to identify refugees who suffer from chronic psychotic illness. You can then manage their illness so that they can stay with their families, continue to work, and spend as little time as possible in hospital.

Even when these people are no longer acutely psychotic, they may continue to act in strange ways. They often seem out of touch with reality. They have strange beliefs that are not true. For example, they may believe they are God

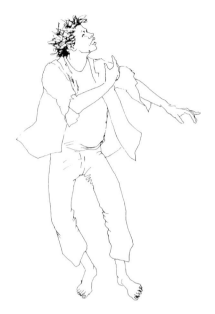

People with chronic psychosis may be called "mad" or "crazy"

or a king. Sometimes they have strong feelings that people are trying to hurt them. Often they hear voices and see or smell things that do not exist. For instance, they may say they are able to hear the voice of a dead ancestor talking to them or about them outside their head. Sometimes they may join in with the talking and seem to be talking to themselves.

In most cultures, people with this illness are unkindly called "mad" or "crazy". Sometimes others will avoid them because they are considered to be possessed, or it is thought they will bring bad luck or are dangerous. However, these people are suffering from a disease of the brain. The cause of this disease is still unknown but treatment can often help them. Refugees who have this illness are not bad people. People with this illness are more likely to be hurt or cheated by others than they are to hurt or cheat others.

The major symptoms of chronic psychosis are:

* false beliefs;

* hearing voices or seeing or smelling things that do not exist;

* speaking very quickly or very slowly;

* talking to oneself or making strange comments to others;

* becoming withdrawn or overly excited;

* bizarre behaviour such as waving hands, shouting, collecting useless things and religious behaviour that is abnormal in one's culture;

* difficulty in sleeping or disturbed sleep;

- becoming easily upset or frightened by intimate relationships and personal responsibilities.

People with this illness often suffer from it throughout their lives.

How to identify people with chronic psychosis

1. Find out if the person has any of the symptoms of a chronic psychotic illness. Ask when the symptoms first started. Has the person ever had to be hospitalized or treated for acute psychosis? What events may have caused these acute episodes or made the symptoms worse? What treatments helped to relieve the symptoms?

2. Make a list of every occasion the person was admitted to hospital and the type of treatment that was given.

3. Make sure you ask the person directly,

   "Do you hear voices when there is no one there?"

   If so, ask, "Do these voices ever tell you to harm yourself or others?"

   If so, ask, "Have they ever told you to kill yourself or anyone else?"

   Decide how dangerous the situation is by finding out if the person is likely to follow the commands given by the voices.

4. Decide whether the person's psychosis is due to depression (see page 42). If it is, treat the depression.

5. Like acute psychosis, chronic psychotic illness can be caused by physical disease. Arrange for those who are psychotic to be examined by a doctor or nurse at the health centre.

6. Find out all the ways in which the psychotic illness has made it difficult for the person to work properly at home, at a job or at school. Ask the family in what ways they would like to see the person improve.

How to help people with chronic psychosis

Make a treatment plan for helping the person over a long period. Your four goals are:

- To keep the person out of hospital by preventing acute psychosis from developing.

- To protect the person from danger.

- To find ways to keep the person busy — working, going to school or helping others.

- To educate the family and community not to be angry, hurtful or abusive. They must be taught that the person has a disease that causes the strange behaviour and actions.

You can achieve these goals in the following ways.

1. Get the person to trust you. People with chronic psychosis may be very suspicious of you. If this is so, discuss the problem openly with the person concerned. Act in a calm and friendly manner.

   Remember, how long you see the person for is not as important as how often. Try to have frequent brief meetings, at least once every week. The person may not be able to bear more than a 15-minute meeting with you. Work together to help the person avoid people and situations that make the symptoms worse.

2. Make a plan to keep the person with chronic psychosis busy. This can be arranged with both the patient and the family. Someone who has nothing to do will get into trouble. Lack of activity may also make the symptoms worse. Find work or activities that the person is able and willing to do.

3. Help the person with chronic psychosis to stop drinking alcohol and using drugs. Drugs and alcohol will make psychotic symptoms worse and more difficult to treat.

4. If the person agrees, speak to senior family members, the employer and religious leaders. Tell them that the person has a disease and needs their support. Suggest simple ways in which they can help. Ask them to tell you immediately if the patient's symptoms get worse so that you can observe and examine them. Observing the symptoms may help you find the cause of the upset and get rid of it. A person who gets worse may require an increase in the dose of medication (see below). A person who is helped before becoming psychotic will not have to be admitted to hospital.

If a medical doctor is available to examine and treat the person:

5. Try to arrange for the person to be given a drug such as haloperidol in doses of 0.5 to 5 mg a day at bedtime. On rare occasions a higher dose may have to be given but look out for the major side-effects of this drug. (For more details see page 47.)

   To avoid these side-effects, trihexyphenidyl may be given in doses of 2 mg in the morning and at bedtime. If there are still major side-effects, it may be necessary to reduce the dose of haloperidol.

6. Always make sure that the person is taking the medicine. If you find out from the person or family that the medication is not being taken, or if you suspect that this is the case, the person could be given an injection of a drug every 2–4 weeks. For example, fluphenazine decanoate could be given in

doses of 25–50 mg into the muscles every 3–4 weeks. Trihexyphenidyl should also be given if the person complains of side-effects (see above).

Remember to make sure that the person you are trying to help is taking the medication. Make sure that only the smallest dose needed to reduce the person's symptoms is given.

Mental disorders caused by hurtful and frightening events

Emotional symptoms may be associated with very hurtful events and terrifying life-threatening situations. These events may be caused by other people, as in the case of torture or imprisonment. They may also be caused by natural disasters such as a severe earthquake with great loss of life. Fortunately, most refugees who have suffered shocking or terrible personal events in their lives do not become mentally ill.

The following are the most common symptoms associated with hurtful, violent and terrifying refugee experiences:

- Flashbacks. The person relives the shocking and hurtful event as if it is happening all over again. For example, people who witnessed the murder of their parents may feel they are witnessing it again just as it actually occurred several months or years before. They hear the sounds, smell the smells and feel the sensations originally associated with the murder. They re-experience this terrifying and hurtful event while awake.

- Continuously remembering the hurtful and terrifying event and not being able to stop thinking about it.

- Nightmares (terrifying dreams).

- Very disturbed sleep.

- Easily getting upset (being shocked by loud noises and sudden sounds such as a door banging or a barrel falling off a truck).

- Feelings of sadness and hopelessness.

- Fear of being left alone or of leaving the house.

- Fear that someone or something is going to hurt one again.

Refugees with these symptoms will usually be exhausted. They will be physically worn out by their daily memories, flashbacks and nightmares. The nightmares wake them up at night and they are so frightened that they cannot go back to sleep. When they get up in the morning, they are tired from lack of sleep and then start having flashbacks and upsetting memories. The cycle is repeated day after day.

Refugees who have this disorder worry a lot and are easily frightened. They fear ordinary things such as the dark, meeting people, or travelling in a car or bus. They often refuse to be left alone. Almost all refugees with this disorder feel hopeless and depressed.

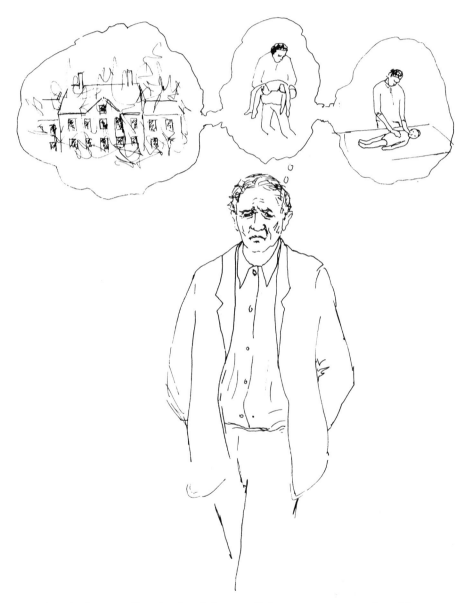

People who have suffered a hurtful or terrifying event may not be able to stop thinking about it

How to identify people with mental disorders caused by hurtful or frightening events

1. Ask the person to tell you of any "hurtful" or "terrifying" experiences. Remember, it is better to ask the refugee a list of direct questions, such as "Did you experience starvation, lack of shelter, torture, imprisonment, murder or deaths in your family?" Do not ask general questions, such as "Have you had a hurtful or terrifying experience?" Find out if any of these terrible events are still occurring.

2. Determine if the refugee has any of the symptoms listed above. Find out how often the symptoms occur. For example, a person may tell you that he or she has nightmares. Ask whether the nightmares are every night, once a week or once a month.

   Remember, many refugees will have some of these symptoms but will not be sick. Only when the symptoms are frequent, severe and exhausting will the person feel ill and seek your help.

3. Find out how much the symptoms interfere with work, school, housework and other activities.

4. Ask specifically about nightmares. Ask for a detailed description of what the person dreams about in the nightmares. The story in the nightmare is almost always the same as the hurtful and terrifying events experienced.

How to help people with mental disorders caused by hurtful or frightening events

The emotional upset associated with hurtful and terrifying experiences can be extremely debilitating. It can be so unpleasant that many refugees with this disorder feel they are "living in hell". You can help in the following ways:

1. Tell people with this kind of disorder that they have an illness and that upsetting memories that keep coming back are part of this illness. Tell them that they must try to push these memories out of their mind. When people are experiencing symptoms do not ask them to talk about their terrible experiences. In the first interview you will already have found out what happened to cause the illness. Asking too many questions about the experience can make people feel worse. At a later stage as they start to feel better they may need to discuss their memories.

2. When rape or sexual violence has occurred, deal with this as suggested in Unit 9, page 126.

3. Tell people with this kind of disorder that, once they feel better, you would like them to tell you about their life — but only if they feel it might be helpful. Then wait for them to share their painful experiences with you.

4. Offer supportive counselling. If members of a divided family wish to be re-united, help them to get back together. Encourage family support.

5. Help people to solve any social or work problems caused by the illness.

6. If appropriate, refer people to religious counsellors or traditional healers to help them understand and accept their tragedy. This may also help them to repair their lives. Remember, religious ritual, ceremonies and practices can have a powerful positive effect on a person suffering from this illness.

If a medical doctor is available to examine and treat patients:

7. Not all people with this kind of disorder need treatment with drugs but some may benefit from it. The sleep disturbance and nightmares may be quickly eliminated by drugs, or traditional herbs and folk remedies, or a combination of both. Medical drugs can also treat the depression which almost always occurs with this illness. Only people with appropriate train-ing and experience should prescribe these drugs.

- Drugs such as imipramine or amitriptyline, in doses of up to 100 mg, may be given at bedtime.

- Watch out for dry mouth, blurred vision and irregular heartbeat, espe-cially if the refugee is known to have heart disease.

- For both drugs, it is best first to offer a 25 mg dose and then to increase it as necessary by 25 mg every few days. These drugs are usually helpful for most symptoms but nightmares may still be troublesome.

- If the nightmares continue, propranolol (10 mg at bedtime), given to-gether with the other medication, may suppress them.

Mental disorders caused by beatings or other injuries to the head

Some refugees may have suffered injury to the head. Some may have experi-enced beatings to the head while being tortured. Others may have had plastic bags placed over their heads or have survived attempts to drown them. Head injury can also occur from shelling or rocket attacks, being thrown from a truck, falling from a height, or sliding down a steep slope.

The brain can easily be damaged by a fall or a beating that might not seem severe to the refugee. After damage on the outside of the head has healed, the refugee may have disabling or unpleasant mental problems.

The following are the most common symptoms of mental disorders caused by beatings or other injuries to the head:

— headaches;

— dizziness;

— tiredness and lack of energy;

— disturbed sleep or loss of sleep;

— arguing or fighting for no reason;

— crying or laughing easily;

— forgetting things easily;

— not being able to pay attention;

— not being able to think clearly;

— worrying in case the mind is "broken";

— no longer being able to work or help with family tasks.

How to identify people with mental disorders caused by beatings or other injuries to the head

Refugees with this problem, or their families, may not be able to recognize a mental illness caused by head injury, especially if the head injury occurred many years ago.

1. Ask all refugees you help if they have been beaten on the head or if they have had other experiences in which the head may have been injured. These could be war injuries, nearly being drowned or nearly suffocating. If so, find out when the event occurred and whether the refugee lost consciousness. If the refugee did lose consciousness, find out how many hours or days or months passed before the person became conscious again. Remember, the longer the refugee was unconscious, the greater the chance of a mental problem related to the event that caused the unconsciousness.

2. Ask questions to test for loss of memory. Ask, for instance, "Do you forget things easily? Are you always being told by your relatives that you are losing things? Do you start to cook food and then forget it is on the stove and burn it?"

3. Find out whether the person who suffered the head injury has noticed a change in behaviour since the injury occurred. Ask the family's opinion too. Is the person easily angered, violent or liable to cry easily? Has the person become difficult to get along with at home or at work? Are family members such as the spouse frustrated or upset? Is this new?

4. Many people who have had a head injury will worry in case their mind or brain is "broken". Find out if they are worrying about this by asking directly, "Do you feel something is wrong with your mind?" If they do feel this way, ask, "What do you think is wrong?"

5. Find out how well the person is able to work and help the family with jobs at home. Interview the husband or wife or other relatives. For example, ask them, "Is your father unable to work or help out at home?" If the answer is "Yes", ask, "Why?"

6. If you decide that a refugee has mental illness due to head injury, it is important to find out whether there are other associated medical or mental illnesses. Find out if the refugee has any medical problems such as fits, severe headaches or inability to use parts of the body. Find out if the person is blind or has trouble in seeing, poor hearing, or strange feelings in the body. These conditions may also have been caused by the head injury. If the person has any of these problems, coordinate the help you give with that of the health centre's doctor or nurse.

7. Examine the refugee for depression (see page 42). Depression will make all the symptoms of head injury worse. If you treat the depression, you will improve most of the symptoms of the head injury.

How to help people with mental disorders caused by beatings or other injuries to the head

Many symptoms caused by head injury cannot be cured completely. This is especially so with symptoms related to remembering and learning new things. But all of the symptoms can be improved. The refugee can also be helped to overcome many of the disabilities associated with this illness.

1. If the person has a depression or any other mental disorder, treat it. This will eliminate or lessen many of the symptoms of head injury.

2. Tell the refugee that he or she has a mental illness due to a head injury. Explain this to the family members too. Tell them you are doing something to help. This will relieve their worry that the refugee's mind is permanently "broken" and that the situation is hopeless.

3. If a refugee who has had a head injury now has chronic headaches, make clear that your treatment of the head injury will help relieve the headaches. Do not focus on the headaches. Do not give any pain relievers stronger than aspirins or paracetamol for the headaches. If treatment of the head injury, including medication for depression, does not relieve the headaches, arrange for a medical doctor or nurse to examine the person again.

4. When people cannot remember things but know how to write, teach them to use a memo pad or notebook.

5. Routine and repetitive tasks should be given to people with these disorders. In this way they will learn a task by doing it again and again.

If a medical doctor is available to examine and treat the person:

6. Medical drugs may be given for anger, temper tantrums and irritability. A person who is not already being treated with an antidepressant may be given amitriptyline or imipramine for depression, starting with 10 mg of either drug once or twice a day. Haloperidol, 1 or 2 mg once or twice a day, can also sometimes control this behaviour.

7. Make sure that people who have fits are treated at the health centre. These people will probably have to take an anticonvulsant medicine such as phenobarbital every day, at least once a day. Sometimes other anti-convulsant medicines have to be taken as often as 3 or 4 times a day.

Emotional disturbances associated with intense fear and worry

Refugees have many worries and fears. They have to cope with many problems they did not have before becoming refugees. These problems may include lack of proper food and shelter, unemployment, and danger from bandits or warfare. Most refugees also think a lot about what they have lost and worry about the future, especially for their children.

Sometimes these worries and fears will overwhelm refugees. An event may occur that is finally too much for them to cope with. They may then develop severe emotional and physical complaints. Neither family nor friends can help relieve these complaints.

A mild depressive illness is often associated with intense fear and worry. The work or school activities of people with such an illness are not seriously disturbed. They will ask for your help only after traditional healers or other medical practitioners have failed to ease their symptoms. They may also have tried drugs and alcohol and found that they have little effect.

The most common mental symptoms of this illness are:

— overwhelming fears and worries;

— muscle aches, soreness, twitching, feeling shaky;

— restlessness, getting easily tired;

— feeling keyed-up or on edge;

— easily being frightened by loud noises or sudden sounds;

— difficulty falling asleep or staying asleep;

— getting angry easily and complaining a lot;

— not being able to keep one's mind on work or play.

The physical symptoms of this illness are:

— rapid and irregular heartbeat;

— shortness of breath;

— sweating or cold clammy hands;

— dry mouth and a lump in the throat;

— dizziness and lightheadedness;

— nausea;

— diarrhoea;

— hot flushes or chills;

— headaches;

— frequent urination;

— impotence or premature ejaculation.

Some people also have special problems such as:

• Fits of fear (or panic), lasting from a few seconds to several minutes. They may include sweating, extreme nervousness, a choking sensation and a feeling that one is going to die or be harmed or go mad.

• A terrible fear of a common object or situation, such as knives, enclosed spaces, open spaces, cats, chickens or other things.

• A terrible fear of leaving home or being in public places.

How to identify people with emotional disturbances associated with intense fear or worry

1. Ask refugees about each of the above symptoms. Compare their major complaints with your list of the most common symptoms of emotional distress in the community. People with these emotional disturbances will have many of the symptoms.

2. Ask, "Who have you already seen for help?" Contact these people. They are usually family elders, traditional healers, priests, doctors or nurses. Find out what they believe may have caused the person's illness and what they did to help.

3. Many physical diseases can cause symptoms similar to those of emotional disturbance. If there is no obvious social or personal cause for the symptoms, a person who has lost weight or does not respond to your help should be sent to a medical doctor or nurse for a physical examination.

4. Find out if the refugee is depressed (see page 42). How serious is the depression?

5. Find out if the refugee has a psychotic illness (see page 46). If so, it is the most likely cause of these symptoms.

6. Find out if the person is using drugs or alcohol to treat these symptoms. Find out how much and for how long.

How to help people with emotional disturbances associated with intense fear and worry

1. Arrange for the medical doctor or nurse to diagnose and treat any physical illnesses, depression, psychosis, and drug and alcohol problems. Give as much help as you can. Give them any information you have and find out how you can help them.

2. Find out which personal and social events and conditions are causing the person's fears and worries. If the person agrees, talk to family, friends, the employer and the religious community about this. Try to persuade them to help the person solve the problems.

3. Do not make promises that you cannot keep. Some problems cannot be solved by anyone, including camp authorities.

4. Traditional healing and religious practices, such as prayer and meditation, can be very helpful. Send the refugee to a traditional healer or priest to see whether they can help, if this has not been tried already.

If a medical doctor is available to examine and treat the person:

5. Fears and worries can sometimes be treated by a medical drug such as diazepam in doses of 5–15 mg 2 or 3 times a day. These drugs may, however, make the person sleepy. The drugs can be dangerous if the person is working with machinery or driving. People can also become dependent on diazepam. Ideally the doctor should give the medication for no longer than one month. A person receiving diazepam should also start immediately with relaxation exercises (see Unit 2). After a few weeks the person will be able to relax and should not need the medication any more.

   Remember that the best solution for this condition is to help refugees solve their own problems, often with help from relatives and friends. If this is impossible, help them live with their problems. Medical drugs cannot do this.

6. Those refugees with fits of panic, fear of common situations or fear of public places may be helped by the drugs used for depression (see page 42).

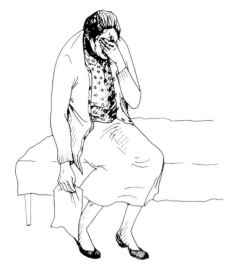

Sleep may be disturbed on receiving bad news about a member of the family

Emotional disturbances related to poor sleep

Almost all refugees have had problems with their sleep. Sleep problems are common to all the mental illnesses you will deal with in your community. Poor sleep can be caused by physical illnesses, especially if there is pain or discomfort. Refugees who abuse drugs or alcohol will also have trouble sleeping.

The most common sleep problems you see will not be caused by illness but by changes in camp conditions. These may include extreme weather conditions such as storms or drought, or worries about new rules related to resettlement, refugee status, food distribution or military activity.

Serious poverty and difficult and unexpected personal situations can also result in poor sleep. For example, a refugee's sleep may suddenly become disturbed on receiving bad news about a member of the family.

Dramatic changes in camp conditions or in a refugee's personal or social situation can turn an occasional sleep problem into a more serious one. The refugee will now sleep badly every night rather than just two or three times a week. The person may also relive the past in bad dreams or worry about the current situation. Lack of sleep and sleep interrupted by bad dreams cause people to feel tired the next day. Eventually a person becomes exhausted by this daily cycle of poor sleep and tiredness.

How to identify people with emotional disturbances related to poor sleep

1. Identify all physical or mental disorders and disturbances that may be causing the refugee's poor sleep. Make sure that the refugee is not depressed. If the person has frequent nightmares, he or she may be suffering from an emotional illness following a hurtful and terrifying event.

2. Find out from the refugee, friends, neighbours and camp authorities if any dramatic changes have occurred in camp life that might worry the person you are trying to help.

3. Ask the refugee and family members when the sleep problem began. Find out what personal or social events may be causing it.

How to help people with emotional disturbances related to poor sleep

1. Treat any medical or mental disorders that may be causing the person's poor sleep. Try to find out about any worries that may be causing the poor sleep.

2. Do not give sleeping tablets to someone with long-standing sleep problems. Although the tablets may help for a few nights, they will not help in the long term. Sleeping tablets may be used for a few nights to help someone who has just been very upset by something, but afterwards they must be stopped.

3. Send the refugee to a priest, religious leader or traditional healer. Folk medicine, prayer, meditation and religious practices can help a great deal.

4. Counsel the refugee about the worries that may be contributing to poor sleep.

5. Help the refugee find a relatively quiet place to sleep. This should be a place where the person feels safe and will not be constantly interrupted by loud noises, children, or people coming into the house or room at all hours of the night. A home visit will help you find out if this is possible.

6. Remember, even with all these measures you may not be able to solve completely the person's sleep problem. You may not be able to improve overcrowded living conditions, poverty or problems with the police or immigration authorities.

7. Some simple things that can be done to help sleep are described in Unit 2, page 28.

Helping refugee children

After studying this unit you should be able to:

1. Understand the special difficulties faced by refugee parents in the artificial environment in which they live.

2. Explain how becoming a refugee changes both culture and child-rearing practices.

3. Understand some ways of protecting the mental health of children and allowing them to develop normally.

4. Recognize particularly vulnerable families and understand how to meet their needs and those of unaccompanied children.

5. Understand the need to keep appropriate records.

Children become refugees when they seek safety with their parents or are sent for safety outside their own country. They may also become refugees by being born to parents who are already refugees. They often find themselves in a culture different from their own.

Many children have traumatic life events but not all have mental health problems. Although only a small proportion of people need mental health care, people who work with refugee children and their families should be able to recognize signs of mental disorder or emotional distress in children and know how to help. Help that is appropriate for refugee children may be different from help that is appropriate for children who are not refugees.

As far as possible, refugee children should be cared for within their families and communities. Child care workers must seek the help of traditional health, religious and social systems to treat children in ways that are appropriate to their culture.

Looking after the mental health of refugee children

Refugee populations can help themselves if they are given the chance to do so. It often used to be thought that refugees needed only to be provided with material needs such as food, water, shelter and medical care. Now we know that refugees must also be helped to recover their emotional, cultural and spiritual strength. Work with children involves meeting both material and nonmaterial needs. Helping the whole refugee community to maintain its mental health will provide great support to children.

Factors that would improve the mental health and well-being of refugee children include:

- A return to the security that a strong and stable family can offer.

- Living in a stable environment which does not change from day to day. Children need goals that are attainable as well as structure and a sense of purpose in their lives.

- Provision of material needs such as food, water and medical care.

- Help for both parents and children in recovering from emotional shocks.

- Experiences that children living "normal" lives might expect. For example, refugee children need positive role models (people who set a good example

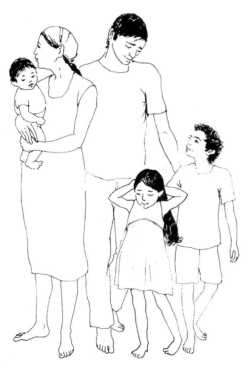

A strong stable family can improve the mental health of children

and whom children can imitate). Like other children, refugee children need to learn new skills and receive education.

- A belief in the future and the opportunity to influence what happens to them.

- Some understanding and acceptance of what has happened to them and why it happened. This could be explained in political or other terms.

- The opportunity to complete all the normal stages of child development.

- The time and opportunity to recover after their experiences and to grieve over the deaths of those they were close to.

Remember, children can benefit from childhood only if they have the support and care necessary for normal psychological development. To deprive a child of that support is as serious as depriving him or her of food and shelter.

The special needs of refugee children

When children and their parents become refugees they face separation, loss, uncertainty, stress and hardship. These can disrupt the normal growth and development of children.

Refugee parents have many difficulties and may themselves suffer as a result of:

— the shock of the events that made them refugees;

— abuse, violence or torture;

— the death of one or more family members;

— witnessing the death, torture, imprisonment or disappearance of family members;

— grief over the loss of country, language, culture, career and property;

— fear for their personal safety now and in the future;

— worry about the safety of family members imprisoned, left behind or separated from them during the journey.

To be a refugee is to live in an artificial environment. Refugees are living neither as they did in the past nor as they will in the future. In a refugee situation the roles of adults and parents become very different. Adults can remember the past, their own childhood and life before the move. Refugee children may have spent their whole lives, or all they can remember of them, as refugees. They may have seen their parents only as refugees and may have few memories of how they were before. Camp life is not a normal way to live.

Refugee life means:

- People may not know what is going to happen to them and have no control over their situation.

- There is very little or no employment.

- There is little space and movement, and not much to eat and drink.

- Normal roles, cultural life and daily routines have been lost, leaving people uncertain, frustrated and depressed.

Because of this situation parents in the camp may become very dependent on having things done for them. They may seem not to bother what happens to them. Men lose their means of earning and providing for their families. Women lose their traditional ways of caring for their families and rearing their children. Everyone loses self-respect, motivation and interest in life.

Building a cultural framework

Culture provides identity and continuity for children. The beliefs and values that hold people together in families and communities are passed on through culture.

Remember:

It is best if those who work with refugee children are from the children's own culture and share the same language. With the help of interpreters, it is usually possible to find paraprofessionals or professionals in the refugee community to do the work. Other members of the refugee community can be trained to take over the work in due course. Look first to the refugee community for workers.

If you are working with refugee children who are not of your culture, you can get help and information about the children's culture from other refugees. When talking to the community you might want to ask how people care for their children, what rituals and celebrations they have, and what hopes they have for the future. Also ask about the roles of different family members. Find out how the community cares for children without families.

Ask about how children are cared for and reared in the refugees' home country:

- Does the immediate family (mother, father, sisters and brothers) care for infants? Or is there an extended family system where grandparents, aunts and uncles care for children?

- Who disciplines children and how do they do it?

- Are certain kinds of behaviour accepted until the child reaches a certain age? Is the child then expected to mature and behave differently?

- Are children from large families often sent to live with other family members? If so, what is the children's role in their new family groups?

- What do parents expect of their children at different ages? What work do parents expect a child of a certain age to do in the home? How much is a child of a certain age expected to look after brothers and sisters? At what age would children normally start school and how long would their education last? When would they learn a trade? When would they leave home?

In particular, ask about care for unaccompanied children:

- What is the traditional way of caring for children without relatives?

- If traditional methods of care are no longer .available, how are children being looked after now?

- What does the community think about foster care (taking responsibility for someone else's child for a period of time), adoption or caring for other people's children?

Changes in child-rearing practices

The child-rearing practices of refugee communities have usually been disrupted. This may not have happened only recently. Child-rearing practices may have been disrupted for a number of years because of troubles in the home country, famine, a series of moves, or losses to the family or the whole community.

Why child-rearing practices change

Child-rearing practices may change because:

- Families may not be able to provide for their children in the way they used to. It may no longer be possible for parents to fulfil their earlier roles.

- Men are unable to work and support the family as before. They may not be able to make decisions about what will happen to their families.

- Women are unable to carry out the daily tasks they used to do for their families.

- Families may no longer get much support from the community. For example, the community may no longer organize religious ceremonies or education for refugee children. Economic events like markets and cultural events like dances or theatre may have stopped.

- Refugee parents often feel powerless to help their children.

- Family roles are changed or lost. The stress of this may lead to family abuse or neglect. The family unit may even break down.

- Refugee families are often headed by single mothers who may have to spend most of their time at work to make sure that the family survives. This can seriously damage the normal mother–child relationship.

All of these things affect the family in general and child-rearing in particular.

How to recognize the mental health problems of children

To recognize children who may have mental health problems, it is necessary to listen and observe. Listen to what children say both in words and through their behaviour. Observe what children do as you talk with them or as they play alone or with others. Later in this unit there are lists of signs of distress in children of different ages.

- Talk with parents and other adults who know the child. Is the child behaving differently from before? Have the child's personality, mannerisms or outlook on life changed greatly? Do the adults think the child needs help?

- Talk to the child about everyday things and observe how the child responds. Does the child listen to you and understand what you are saying? Does the child's understanding seem satisfactory for its age?

- Does the child appear very confused or upset? Is he or she unable to concentrate or respond to questions?

- Compare the child's behaviour with that of other children in the same setting. Is it about the same as the behaviour of other refugee children in the camp? Do children in this camp appear to have about the same behaviour and interests as local children?

- Observe the child at play. Does the child play appropriately for his or her age? Is the playing typical of other children or is it somehow different?

If you find that a child has a mental health problem, question the parents or other carers to find out if the problem was there before or if it has started recently and seems to be a result of recent events in the child's life.

If the problem was present before, the treatment will differ. Also, an existing problem is likely to be made worse by the disruption of becoming a refugee.

Problems that occur because someone is a refugee are more likely to improve as a result of help given to the family and child. Some of the ways of helping children of different ages and their mothers are discussed in the following sections.

Helping young children and mothers

Identifying infants who need special help

Look out for the following signs of mental distress and problems in a child under 2 years of age:

- The child cries all the time or gets hysterical (crying wildly and screaming).

- The child shows little interest in what is happening or is frightened of people who come near. This may be due to malnutrition, not enough emotional care or, more often, a combination of the two.

- The child has difficulty in eating or sleeping.

- The child bangs his or her head or rocks backwards and forwards.

- There is no "babbling" or "baby talk".

- The child is unresponsive. This may be because the child is not getting enough physical contact (is not being held or touched enough).

- The child returns to the behaviour of a much younger infant (for example, the child may stop walking or trying to talk).

- The child may be late in beginning actions such as smiling, sitting, walking or talking. Remember, however, that babies do not all develop at the same rate.

All these signs can result from malnutrition or lack of maternal care, or both. There is often a damaging cycle — the less responsive a child is, the easier it is to overlook his or her needs. This is especially true when there are older children who also need attention. Babies that we say are "good babies" because they are quiet and unresponsive may in fact be showing the effects of serious malnutrition or neglect.

Infants with mental health problems may have delayed development. Delays may have psychological or physical causes, including malnutrition. In both cases the treatment is the same: provide mother and child with an infant stimulation programme.

Helping mothers to stimulate their infants

"Stimulation" means actively encouraging infants to use:

— their senses (sight, hearing, etc.);

— their motor abilities (their skills in moving);

— their ability to learn and to solve problems;

— their ability to communicate with others.

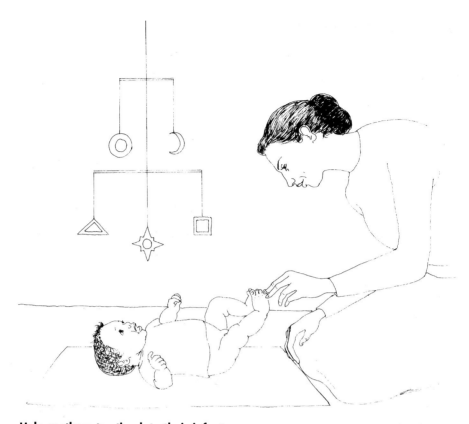

Help mothers to stimulate their infants

The aim of stimulation is to maintain the infant's development or to help the infant come as close as possible to the normal level of development. This is important for two reasons. First, stimulation motivates the baby physically. Second, it encourages the baby to make contact with the mother or carer. Mother and child respond to this attention. Their relationship becomes stronger. The mother can start to feel in control of at least one part of her life. She can see the immediate positive result in the baby. The mother is pleased, so the baby wants to do more.

This attachment to the mother is one of the most important steps in child development. From this early experience of trust and love, children learn communication skills that they will use for the rest of their lives.

Ways to stimulate speech

The mother can do the following to help to stimulate speech:

- Talk to the infant while breast-feeding or spoon-feeding. Make eye contact and talk or sing to the infant while nursing.

- Put the infant on her lap or hold it in front of her as she talks. Name parts of the body or objects and sing and tell stories.

- Carry the infant around with her and name objects. Talk about the surroundings or what she is doing. Tell the child where she is going.

This type of stimulation can have the following results:

- The mother conveys a sense of caring and warmth through the direct contact and attention she gives to the child.

- Older infants become more aware of their surroundings.

- The child has an opportunity to hear words and learn how they are formed as the mother says them again and again.

- The infant begins to attach words and names to objects and activities.

- Older infants form the basis of a vocabulary.

Infant stimulation does not need to be dealt with in a complicated programme. Often mothers have very little time to attend sessions outside the home.

Other helpful activities

- Help the family to construct or find a few simple playthings and encourage mother and child to play together for short periods every day.

- Get older children or relatives to play with or stimulate the baby using the toys at hand.

- Make toys from local materials. Making toys can be another way to involve parents in caring for the child.

- Folk stories and songs should always be part of activities with children.

- Search for items an infant would play with under normal circumstances.

Using play to stimulate young children

Here are some suggestions of simple playthings that can be used to stimulate infants as they play.

Plaything	Activity and purpose
Traditional toys made by parents	Encourages parents to be involved with the child when he/she plays.
Small stones in a gourd or plastic container	Used as a rattle to encourage the baby to listen to, look for and find the sound.
Larger stones and a gourd	Stones are put into and taken out of gourd to help eye–hand coordination.
Doll/animal figure made of cloth	Teaches the child to recognize figures. The child can touch, taste and handle the figure in play.
Soft ball of tightly rolled cloth	Rolled back and forth between the adult and child to improve eye–hand coordination. This also helps the child to play with other people.
Bright objects hung up as a mobile over the child's bed	If they are placed out of reach, the baby will look at the objects, follow them with its eyes and reach for them.

Stimulating infants with malnutrition, illness or delayed development

Young children recovering from severe malnutrition, illness or delayed development need activities that encourage them to use their bodies. Here are some examples:

- Instead of handing a plaything to a child, hold the plaything so the child reaches up to get hold of it.

- Place an object just out of reach of the child so that he or she has to move to get it. Then place it a short distance away so the child has to crawl to reach it.

- Find a suitable place where infants learning to walk have something to hold on to and can pull themselves up onto their feet if they fall. Make a frame for infants to hold on to. Place a toy where the child can reach it by standing up.

- If an infant is able to stand, encourage him or her to step away from the frame towards the mother. The mother should wait ready to receive the child.

- Do not rush the activities. Young children who have not been active need time to learn to use their bodies and to become confident enough to try to do new things.

- Do not move a toy out of an infant's reach too often. This will frustrate and discourage the infant from trying again. Give the child a chance to reach and hold the toy.

- Always look for activities that make the child look, listen, reach for things, talk to people and think about what is happening.

- A baby's contact with the mother (looking at each other, being talked to and making sounds) is as important as playing.

Help or encourage mothers to do these types of activities with their young children. Work with mothers individually or in small groups.

Stimulating infants in groups

All the above stimulating activities for infants can be carried out in groups as well as by mothers on their own with their children. You may wish to organize meetings of groups of mothers and young children. Here are some things to remember when you set up a group like this.

- Each group should include no more than six or eight mothers with their children.

- The group should be led by a person who has a basic knowledge of child development and of group work with mothers. The leader should come to all group sessions and should get along well with the mothers. In time, members of the group can be trained to start their own groups.

- Meetings should be held in a quiet place without onlookers. There should be space for mothers and children to move around.

- Meetings should be held in the cool of the morning before the children or adults are tired.

- The group should meet at least three times and up to five or six times. Sessions should last one hour and should be held at least once a week.

- Mothers should be told the number of times the group will meet and how often and at what time sessions will be held.

Mothers who need special help

If a mother is severely depressed by her situation, you may decide that it is necessary to arrange for more support than a group can offer. It is still best not to move the mother and child from the home, if possible. Here are some ways to offer support:

- Arrange home visits to make sure that the mother and child have lots of support to begin with. As the mother gets better, visits can be decreased gradually.

- It may be possible to get relatives, neighbours or other women who are alone to help in the day-to-day care of the mother and child.

- Later a group of home visitors of this kind should be trained to keep an eye on the mother and child.

- In very extreme cases, it may be necessary to move the child and mother to a place where they can be cared for. Mother and child must not be separated.

Helping the preschool child

After a young child stimulation programme, it is important to continue with programmes for older preschool children. This is a very good way of preventing refugee children from falling behind in their development. Stimulation programmes may be linked with organized preschool groups. Refugee children may never have had the opportunity for such an experience before. They may never have been able to use the materials normally found in a preschool, like paper, scissors, paints and clay. This is an important experience in children's development and it helps to prepare them for school.

Preschool groups give parents a few hours away from the demands of the young child. More importantly, preschool groups offer a safe care arrangement if parents have to be away from home during the day. You may have to find children whose parents cannot look after them during the day. In some cultures children are left in the care of an older child and the idea of taking a young child to a preschool group at a set time may seem unusual. You may have to explain and discuss this idea with parents to make it work.

Identifying children of between two and four years who need special help

Preschool children in special need of stimulation may have a number of symptoms. Here are some typical symptoms to look for in children needing special attention:

- The child seems to be going back to an earlier stage of development. For example, the child may act like a younger child in speaking or in controlling his or her behaviour.
- The child sucks its thumb or fingers.
- The child wets the bed at night or wets itself in daytime even though it has already been toilet-trained.
- The child loses control over its bowels.
- The child has nightmares and night terrors.
- The child is frightened of real or imagined objects.
- The child is hyperactive or behaves in a way that the family cannot control.
- The child is aggressive towards others.
- The child shows obvious fear and mistrust of others.

- The child is unable to concentrate.
- The child is not active at all or is unresponsive.
- The child has difficulties in learning.

Stimulating the preschool child

Whether you are helping preschool children within the family or in preschool groups, it is important to know which activities are appropriate for this age group.

Speech activities

Preschool children understand that language and words are for communicating what they want. During the preschool years they spend a lot of energy practising and perfecting words and learning how to use them.

Increase the child's chances of using these new skills of talking. Look for ways to introduce new words and their meanings.

Most important, continue to set aside special time to talk to the children face to face and to listen to them, even if for only a few minutes a day. In preschool groups, children learn to sit in circles for songs and word games. They may not be able to do it when you first start the group, but this is the beginning of learning how.

Play activities

Here are some suggestions of toys that can help stimulate preschool children as they play.

Toys	Pebbles, clay shapes, beads or sticks.
Activity	Children sort them by size, colour and shape.
Purpose	Develops a systematic way of classifying things. This early concept of groups and categories is the first step to organizing and counting.
Toys	Play objects or implements for things that adults do, such as sweeping, gardening or writing. An activity may not require a toy but just an adult with the time to lead an imaginary game.
Activity	Let children "help" with your work in simple tasks such as carrying water or food and cleaning at home. Join in when the child wants to imitate what you do. Explain what you do each day and why.
Purpose	This is the age of imitative play. By such play children learn what adults do and start to establish their own identity. More importantly, it is a first step in learning more serious concepts of right and wrong, moral and social obligations and how adults treat one another.

Continued

Toys	Objects for small hand skills: paper for tearing into shapes or cutting; pencils and crayons for drawing and colouring; sticks for drawing in the earth; beads (of paper or clay) for stringing together; cups or gourds for pouring back and forth water, sand, gravel or mud; simple sewing materials. Objects for large skills: hoops and sticks for rolling; balls for kicking and throwing (can be cloth, wooden or woven) or even tin cans for kicking; swings (from cloth hammocks or carrying slings); climbing frames or sliding boards (from wood, tin or bamboo).
Activity	For small skills, practise with the toys, draw pictures or make things. For large motor skills, play games that involve running, skipping, throwing and kicking (usually alone as preschool children are not yet old enough for group sports).
Purpose	Improves coordination between eye and hand and overall body coordination at an important time. As with speech, there is a long period of development during which all these skills are practised and repeated. Self-esteem and self-confidence improve when skills are mastered. Learning skills encourages independence and gives the child courage to try new things.

Group activity

With their mothers, preschool children can sit in a circle and begin to listen to songs, or learn them, and play word games. This helps with speech. Songs with hand or body movements (ritual folk dances) help with coordination and rhythm. Group work is the start of learning to work with others.

Helping children of school age

The years during which children are normally at school are important for their development. Their view of the world and what happens in it changes dramatically during this time.

Identifying children of school age who need special help

Children of school age (6–11 years) in need of special attention for stimulation may have some of the following symptoms:

- The child may be always crying.

- The child may tremble or appear frightened.

- The child may indulge in self-stimulation such as rocking back and forth or banging the head.

- The child may have sleep disorders, nightmares or sleeplessness, or may sleep excessively.

- The child may wet the bed.

- The child may have eating disorders.

- There may be physical illnesses or problems such as headaches, dizziness, backaches, eye strain or stomach upsets with no apparent cause.

- The child may be physically aggressive or very loud and rough during play.

- The child may be extremely withdrawn, quiet and well-behaved, never expressing feelings or desires, or depressed and unresponsive.

- The child may start acting like a much younger child (for example, there may be loss of bladder control).

- There may be restlessness and inability to complete a task.

- The child may be unable to concentrate or remember things in school.

- The child may be irritable towards others or unable to work with others.

- The child may be frightened of others and unable to trust them.

- The child may be always thinking that bad things will happen in the future.

Stimulating children of school age

If a child's disturbances are not severe, even the simple step of parents or care-giver listening sympathetically may help. If more help is needed, one way of doing this is to provide opportunities for play or other activities that help children relieve their own stress and anxiety.

How play helps

Play is a way of relaxing and interacting with other children for enjoyment. It requires very little involvement from adults. It is also a way of developing physical, mental, emotional and social skills.

Children can express their feelings through drawing, painting, making things or doing drama activities. In this case an adult who knows the children and is a sensitive listener can help them to express their feelings.

Play provides a way for children to talk about their feelings and what has happened to them following a disturbing event. This special healing use of play requires the help of a child specialist or someone skilled in working with children in this way.

How groups help

Children with mental health problems may also be helped by meeting in groups. Groups are an important part of working with children of school age. An adult leads the group and it can have different goals and activities according to the needs of the children.

Groups offer structure, consistency, security and a safe place to learn. They offer stability in the familiar form of an event with a beginning, middle and end. This may sound simple but it is an important source of security to a child.

Groups allow children to see others with similar feelings and problems. Children see how others react to problems and learn the steps in solving problems.

Activities in groups take place in a structured setting where children know the rules and know what is expected of them.

Types of children's groups

Some children's groups may meet just for recreation. "Recreation" means simple games, sports and structured play activities that children would be playing in normal circumstances. Materials do not need to be elaborate and, wherever possible, parents and adults from the community should be involved in the preparation and running of such activities.

Activity groups with a focus are also beneficial. Find adults in the community to teach children folk or cultural arts such as dances, songs and drama. This would normally happen but in the refugee setting it may need to be specifically organized. If it is already taking place in the camp it may only need some material assistance such as the construction of a shelter or provision of some simple equipment. Activity groups may also focus on other forms of expression such as drawing, painting, clay modelling, music, singing and stories. Cultural activities strengthen cultural ties and provide a routine for children. Folk songs, dances and stories are familiar to the community and comforting to the children.

Groups that provide some level of treatment follow naturally from activities that allow children to express themselves better. Children who are unable to talk about their problems can be helped to express their fears through drawing, music and drama. This requires the help and support of a sympathetic adult trained to listen to and support children.

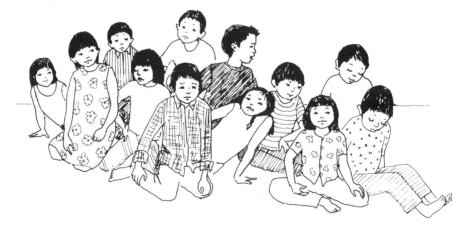

Groups offer children a structure, consistency, security and a safe place to learn

Groups for refugee children

- Children's groups should be well structured and stable.

- Groups should meet once or twice a week and should last for about one hour.

- Groups should always meet at the same time and do what has been agreed.

- There should normally be 4–6 members, but no more than 12.

- Children should be allowed privacy and confidentiality.

- Groups should meet in a calm, private place with no curious onlookers or parents watching.

- Group leaders should be prepared to discuss with the parent and child, in a separate meeting, what has gone on in the group.

- Groups should create an atmosphere of security and safety so that children can express their needs.

The mental health needs of young people aged 12–18 years

The main problems of people in this age group relate to separating from their families and becoming independent. It is important for their development that they are able to practise skills with other young people of the same age.

They also need to copy adult behaviour as they gradually take on adult roles in their community and society. The passage from childhood to adulthood is vital to healthy development.

Symptoms of distress in young people include:

— withdrawal from others; failure to form relationships;

— identifying too much with others; being dependent on others for direction;

— aggressive behaviour, attitude or actions;

— agitation, restlessness or inability to remain still or concentrate;

— extreme depression; unresponsiveness to the extent that they are immobile (catatonic);

— moodiness or changes of mood and behaviour from one extreme to another in a short time;

— functional or physical complaints (such as frequent headaches, stomach upsets, eye strain) caused by stress (see Unit 2);

— sleep problems;

— hallucinations; seeing or hearing things that do not exist;

— paranoia or inability to trust others; feeling that others are threatening to do harm;

— suicide attempts.

The refugee situation can make matters worse because:

— young people are prematurely separated from family because of forced movements or poverty;

— young people's roles in the community and the community itself may change;

— family needs may force young people into adult roles earlier than is normal.

Three common problems

In work with refugee children there are three common problems that cause special concern and require extra attention.

Firstly, some children belong to vulnerable families. These families need to be identified because they are liable to family breakdown. They should be given help to prevent family breakdown from happening.

Secondly, many children may be unaccompanied. They have special needs. If these needs are not met, serious mental health problems are likely to occur. Grief over loss of family and home is normal and the child must be allowed — and even encouraged — to talk about this loss.

Thirdly, the mental health records of children need very careful attention. They should reflect the culture in which the child has been reared. They must also remain confidential. Mental health records should not include information that could be used to threaten or harm the child or the child's family.

Vulnerable families

In any emergency there are three particularly vulnerable kinds of family:

— single-parent families, especially those with several small children;

— large families;

— families that are caring for other people's children in addition to their own.

It is important to identify vulnerable families early. Find them by:

— interviewing new arrivals at registration points, food distribution centres, health care centres or other places where people gather;

— conducting house-to-house surveys;

— asking refugee leaders to identify families with problems;

— contacting relief organizations which may already have identified such families.

Why parents may abandon children

Parents may reach the point of abandoning children if they feel that their situation is desperate. For instance:

- The parents are unable to care for all the children in their care.

- The parents do not have enough water, food, fuel or other materials and see no help coming.

- The parents are discouraged and uncertain about the future and their ability to care for their children.

- The parents are ill or in poor health, malnourished and have no hope. This means that, physically and mentally, they are not able to care for their children.

- One or more of the children is in poor health and is not recovering.

Help for vulnerable families

The right type of help delivered in the right way can keep vulnerable families together. Help can be given both in the short term and in the long term.

Examples of short-term help

- Providing material items.

- Medical care.

- Extra feeding.

- Stimulation programmes for children.

- Training of adults in parenting skills.

Examples of long-term help

- Agricultural help, including land and livestock, for rural families.

- Work training, small business loans and day care for urban families.

- Improvement of the community as a whole.

- Child care arrangements.

- Eventual help to return to the home country.

Unaccompanied children[1]

Family breakdown and separations are often inevitable in mass movements of people. They are especially likely if the situation in the refugee camp is unstable.

Emergency care for unaccompanied children should provide for immediate needs, including shelter, food, medical care, a stable environment, and physical and emotional security. At the same time, information must be collected about each child and about missing family members. A tracing centre should be set up where information can be collected and made available to children seeking their parents or to parents seeking their children.

Early in an emergency situation, pay special attention to young children and infants. It is important to make sure that their health, nutrition and development needs are met.

- There should be a medical examination for each child and medical records must be kept.

- Each child should be immunized (vaccinated) against measles, especially infants aged between 6 months and 5 years.

- Each child should be given vitamin A in the correct dose for the child's age.

- Children should be screened for malnutrition, especially those under 6 years of age. Those found to have nutritional deficiencies should be referred to feeding centres.

- Each child should be screened for psychological problems and delayed development caused by malnutrition, poor health, disease or neglect.

In the longer term, the care given should be appropriate to the child's age and culture. Care should resemble as closely as possible what would be provided in a natural family situation. The care given to unaccompanied children should aim to meet a range of needs.

- **Physical needs.** Children need adequate food, water, shelter, clothing and sanitary conditions to maintain good physical health.

- **Medical needs.** Medical services must be provided for medical emergencies and other illnesses as well as for immunization.

---

[1] The UNICEF manual *Assisting in emergencies* describes the administrative management of unaccompanied children and also touches on their emotional and developmental needs. The manual was published by UNICEF in New York in 1986. A revision is in preparation.

- **Psychological needs.** All people, and particularly young children, have emotional needs. It is essential for children's present and future well-being to provide them with a stable and secure environment. Unaccompanied children must be enabled to maintain an affectionate long-term relationship with an adult. Children need to be able to speak the same language as those around them and stay within their ethnic community or culture. They also need help with individual needs and difficulties.

- **Special needs.** Unaccompanied children should receive the same level of material help as the rest of the refugee population. They should have the same type of housing, the same food, and the same use of the camp school, medical centre and other facilities. Unaccompanied children should not be helped to a higher standard of living, however, for this may tempt vulnerable families to abandon children in order to get more material aid. In difficult circumstances, when there is a threat to physical safety and the future is uncertain, parents may encourage children to leave them and enter facilities for unaccompanied children. They do this to keep their children safe and to make sure that the children have education, food and opportunities for the future.

The care needed can be provided in several ways:

- Each child may be assigned to an appropriate adult carer.

- Unaccompanied children may be given care in extended families or with other children in small groups. The members of these groups should be from the same culture and, if possible, the same community.

- Trained carers may look after small groups of children.

- Supervised independent living facilities may be provided for older adolescents.

Symptoms of loss

All children who are upset by separation and the loss of their family show similar signs of suffering. Their development may stop and may even seem to reverse.

Infants and toddlers who are separated from their families may often:

— cry intensely for short periods;

— be reluctant to accept the substitute carers;

— refuse food;

— suffer digestive upsets;

— have sleeping problems.

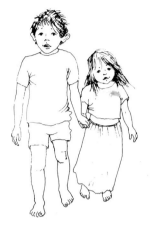

Unaccompanied children have special psychological needs

Children of about 4–5 years may have the same reactions. Also their development may seem to go into reverse. They often behave as they did when they were younger. A child of this age may:

— suck its thumb;

— wet the bed;

— have difficulty controlling impulses (losing its temper easily or acting out other feelings);

— go back to talking as it did when it was younger.

Unaccompanied children aged 4–5 years may often have nightmares and night terrors. They may also be afraid of specific objects or other things (loud noises, animals) and of imaginary beings such as ghosts and witches.

Children of school age can become:

— withdrawn from carers;

— depressed;

— irritable;

— restless;

— unable to concentrate;

— disruptive at school;

— withdrawn from children of the same age.

Adolescents react to separation from their families by becoming:

— depressed;

— moody;

— withdrawn;

— aggressive;

— prone to frequent headaches, stomach pains and other functional complaints.

Providing help to unaccompanied children

Children living without their families and in difficult conditions have lost the special attention they received in their families. Their sense of belonging has gone and with it the assurance that they could rely on the family in all circumstances.

This loss, together with bereavement and the process of grieving that needs to take place, can greatly affect a child's behaviour. Whether mental health problems occur immediately or years later, the loss of the family can seriously disturb the functioning of the child or young adult, even to the extent of being unable to carry on with daily life.

In providing psychological help to unaccompanied minors who have lost their parents, experience has shown that one of the greatest aids to recovery is reunification with family members. The re-establishment of a link to the family, even in the continued absence of parents, can give the child hope for the future and a sense of security and belonging.

If there is no reunion, it is important to involve the child in trying to trace the family. This stimulates hope and gives the child self-esteem associated with active participation in the search. This may help to lessen some of the guilt feelings that often overwhelm children who are separated from their parents.

The unaccompanied child must be permitted and encouraged to express grief and sadness at the loss of family, friends, possessions, language, culture and homeland. The ways in which grief is expressed and recovery from grief takes place depend on the culture in which the child has been reared. Often children are not allowed the necessary time and conditions for this process to take place. This can result in serious setbacks in development at the time or even years later.

Younger children need the positive experience of attachment to adult carers. Many refugee children experience a series of losses that include parents and other adult relatives. They then find it difficult to form a close relationship with other adults because they are afraid of experiencing yet another loss. To help them overcome this fear the adult carer needs to have patience. Over a long period of time, the children must be provided with the sense that they are loved.

Mental health records of children

The camp administrator is responsible for keeping records of the health care given to unaccompanied children. The United Nations High Commissioner for Refugees (UNHCR) has produced guidelines on this topic (see "Notes for camp administrators", below).

Do not give children or adults diagnostic labels. Just describe the behaviour and how frequently it occurs. For example, if you think that a child is "very depressed", do not record this as a term, or label, in the records. Simply give a description of the child's behaviour, such as: "Child A is often seen crying during the day, shows no interest when asked to take part in activities with others, and sleeps very badly at night. This has been going on for two weeks."

If you think that a child is suffering from acute anxiety, use a description such as: "Child B cannot concentrate or sit still in school, sleeps badly and eats very little. She asks many questions about the immediate future and refuses to talk about her past experiences. She has been like this the two months she has been here". This tells much more than saying that a child is "depressed" or "abnormal".

As with adults, it is unwise to label children with mental diagnoses, since these may stay with them for the rest of their lives. It is better just to describe their behaviour and say how long they have been like that.

Notes for camp administrators

Record-keeping[1]

Records must be kept for all children who receive health care, whether for physical or psychological problems. Normally only medical treatment and immunization are recorded. Parents may be given copies of the records which they can take with them if they move from one place to another.

In the case of unaccompanied children, record-keeping may be more complicated. Records should include a family history and the findings of interviews with the child. These can be used later in tracing and reuniting families. Details of treatment and care and of the child's progress should also be recorded. Record-keeping may seem a minor aspect of child care but it needs to be done carefully to guarantee confidentiality and to protect the child's rights and interests.

---

[1] Full details about keeping records on unaccompanied children can be found in: Williamson J, Moser A. *Unaccompanied children in emergencies: a field guide for their care and protection.* Geneva, International Social Service, 1987. The text here is summarized from this publication.

Confidentiality

Information should always be recorded carefully and kept safely. Sometimes there are political reasons to avoid recording information about children's relatives. Certain information may become dangerous to the child or to other family members in another place. Sometimes even names and places must be kept confidential. When a family has to move suddenly there is always a risk that records may be lost or leave the hands of the people who made them.

Transfer of information

If it is necessary to transfer medical records or family information to another person or organization, the family should be informed of any risks involved and should be asked if they are happy about the transfer. It is best to use a simple system of cross-references and to label files with numbers or letters. Keep the list of names separate and confidential.

Accuracy in details

Accuracy is essential. In an emergency situation there may be only one chance to interview a family or others who have information about a separated child. All names of people and places should be recorded in the language, script and characters used by the people affected by the emergency. A mis-spelled name could delay and confuse the tracing of a family member.

Unaccompanied children

A record card of key information should be readily available on all children separated from their parents. This should have all the usual details plus extra information about the family. Records of family histories, with family relationships noted, are also important. Family histories are details of the child's past movements and of family members before the child was separated from them. The child, and any brothers and sisters, must be interviewed to find out basic information and to build up details of the child's history.

Records on unaccompanied children

Records on unaccompanied children should include the following information:

- Personal details (with a clear photograph).

- The circumstances in which the child was found (where, by whom, in what situation).

- The circumstances of the separation from the parents (how it happened, where).

- The history of the child before and after the separation from the parents.

- Medical and health records (immunization, growth charts).

- Details of current care and the child's development.

One mistake often made in record-keeping is the use of a psychiatric "label" to refer to emotional problems or behaviour. Accurate diagnosis is very difficult in unsettled refugee conditions. Often what a Western-trained mental health professional sees as psychotic or abnormal behaviour may in fact be normal in the culture of the refugee (e.g. believing one can see a relative who has died). Problems may occur in reaction to situational stress. It is important for the child, the family and future users of the records to avoid the use of labels and one-word terms to describe children or their behaviour.

UNIT 6

Traditional medicine and traditional healers

Learning objectives

After studying this unit, you should be able to:

1. Recognize the various kinds of traditional practitioner with whom you may need to work.

2. Build cooperation with traditional practitioners.

3. Choose traditional practitioners to work with you.

4. Discourage quacks and dangerous traditional practices.

5. Encourage the use of traditional treatment of the mentally ill when it is helpful and discourage it when it is harmful or dangerous.

Most refugees and displaced populations come from areas where the majority of people still use traditional medicine and only a few have access to scientific medical care. Most refugees have never had a medical examination or taken modern medical drugs. They are often afraid of being treated in a way they are not accustomed to. Such people often misunderstand Western medical care. For example, when a child who has been vaccinated too late against measles actually gets measles and dies of the disease, some people may think that the death has been caused by the vaccine. If so, they will strongly oppose any further vaccination.

Many people feel safer if they are treated by their traditional healers in a way they are used to than if they go to hospital. However, although some diseases can be treated in a traditional way, others can be cured only by scientific medicine. It is not wise to fight against traditional healers because most people trust them and seek their advice or care. The best way to help people is to cooperate with traditional healers rather than make them your enemies. The healers will trust you if you trust them. Also, the people you want to help will trust you more if their healers trust you. They will be happier to accept you if you cooperate with their traditional healers.

If you work closely with traditional healers, you will see that they are able to treat many problems and illnesses. They can often relieve physical or mental

89

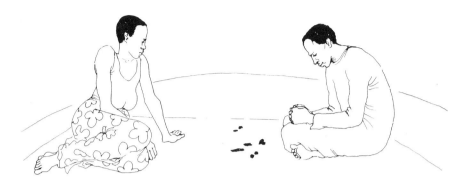

Traditional healers can often relieve physical and mental suffering

suffering, but they cannot deal with all problems. Sometimes scientific medicine can help when they cannot. Work together to find the best way to help people.

Remember that refugees and displaced people will usually go back to their homes eventually. When they do, they may no longer be able to benefit from scientific medicine. They may have to rely on traditional healers in the future.

The different kinds of traditional practitioner

Each society has different kinds of traditional healer. Generally there are six kinds, in addition to traditional birth attendants who deliver babies and advise on the care of mother and child. The six general types of traditional healer are described here although some may use methods from more than one of the categories.

- Some traditional healers first listen to people's complaints and then ask questions about their symptoms. Then they prescribe a medication made from plants or other substances or give other kinds of physical treatment. Although such healers do not make a physical examination, they work in a similar way to medical doctors. They are useful to work with.

- Other traditional healers seek the nature of the illness and its cure by meditating or going into a trance in order to get advice from a god or spirit. They claim that their knowledge comes from a divinity. The treatment may be a certain kind of plant, to be collected under certain circumstances. It could also be an offering to a particular spirit or god, or a special diet. These healers often predict how the illness will progress and what will happen to the sick person. It may not be easy to work with these healers because they have no obvious place in a modern health team, but you can try. In any case, stay on good terms with them and do not stop people from seeking their help.

- In some cultures, people believe that each person has a fixed number of souls. These souls may leave the body and wander around, especially at night when people dream. A soul may get lost and be unable to find its way back, and this is why a person becomes sick. A person with special powers, called a "shaman" in some cultures, will try to find the soul and return it to the body of the sick person. The shaman often goes into a state of trance. The ritual may last for several hours or days. Usually, shamans practise in the house of the person who has sought their help or in their own premises. They may also be allowed to practise in the hospital wards. This can be a good thing because it may prevent people from leaving the hospital to seek their help.

- Some traditional healers use magic as a cure because they believe that illnesses have supernatural origins. They think that illnesses are caused by spirits that have been offended and are seeking revenge, or by black magic sent by other people. Some people believe that a spirit can be introduced by black magic into another person's body. They believe that this spirit can cause physical or mental problems. Healers who use magic make their diagnoses in many different ways. Depending on the person seeking help and the culture, healers use very different rituals to counteract black magic. Some of the rituals may be useful for treating psychological suffering. You may be able to work with these healers. They can help solve many psychological problems and can treat some mental disorders.

- People who feel sick or uncomfortable in body or mind may consult fortune-tellers. Fortune-tellers give advice and usually say how long it will take for the person to get better. This may help people to keep up hope when life is hard but it may also make things worse if people are told they will never recover. Fortune-tellers use different ways of finding out about what is happening and what is going to happen. Sometimes they may even go into a trance to do this.

  You may find it hard to work with fortune-tellers because it is difficult to know what they will say to people, but on the whole they probably do no harm. People believe what they want or need to believe. You can try to work with them, although this may be frustrating. Never stop people consulting them.

- Some traditional practitioners — men and women — and traditional birth attendants specialize in traditional massage. Traditional massage usually focuses on arteries, veins, nerves, joints and other specific parts of the body rather than on the muscles. The healers use their fingers and thumbs, but also sometimes their feet, and they press hard. This may be useful for the relief of pain and tension but the effects may not last long.

  Experts in massage can be very useful in treating headache or migraine and sometimes body pain. Many people complain of pain in some part of the body even though there is no physical basis for the pain. They are suffering in their mind but feel pain in their body. They often feel better after traditional massage. (See Unit 1 for more explanation of physical pain as a result of social or emotional difficulties.)

How to build cooperation with traditional practitioners

- *Show traditional healers that you respect them.* Traditional healers are respected by their own people. If you do not respect them, they will feel offended and you cannot expect their full cooperation. If the people see that you respect their healers, they will understand that you care about fitting into their society. This way you will gain respect and credibility.

Do not try to prove that scientific medicine is better than traditional medicine. Traditional and scientific medicine complement each other; they do not compete against each other. Sometimes one gives better results than the other. Sometimes the results are the same. In some cases it is useful to use both at the same time. Many people feel much better when they see that nothing is neglected in trying to make them well again.

You will probably find it difficult to persuade the traditional healers and the people who use scientific medicine to use both types of medicine at the same time. They will say that they fear that one will have a bad effect on the other. Tell them that it is better to try than to be afraid for no proven reason.

- *Do not challenge traditional healers.* When you first meet them, many traditional healers will tell you that they can treat all kinds of diseases, especially some diseases for which there is no known cure. Do not argue with them. Do not tell them that this is not possible or that they are lying. You would offend them and perhaps force them into taking risks to prove the value of their treatment. Listen to them. If you have the right attitude they will stop speaking like this when they know you better.

- *Be humble and tolerant.* If you are trained in scientific medicine, admit that there are things it cannot do. It cannot cure all diseases. Traditional healers will find it easier to recognize what they can and cannot do, without being afraid of losing face, if you first admit that scientific medicine sometimes cannot help. Since both types of medicine have their good points, cooperation is wise.

- *Know the difference between genuine traditional healers and quacks.* "Quacks" are unscrupulous people who may know something about traditional healing but are not traditional healers. They often do spectacular but controversial things in order to become famous and make money. They can be very harmful to the people who seek their help and they give traditional healing a bad name. Be careful to work with genuine traditional

92

healers and not with quacks. Support the genuine healers and tell the authorities about the quacks if they are putting the health of the people they treat in danger.

How to choose traditional healers to work with you

Doctors, nurses and missionaries have often opposed traditional healers and tried to stop their practices. Because of this, people in the refugee community may tell you that there are no traditional healers among them. They want to protect their healers. The healers also may be afraid to talk to you. Reassure them that you do not wish to stop them working among their people.

- Explain to the community leaders and the people why you wish to cooperate with the traditional healers. Tell them what your intentions are. Say that you want to help the healers so that they can use their skills for treating people. Say that you think that both traditional and scientific medicine are good and can get along well together.

- Ask to meet several healers, not just one. Tell them about your plans and how you would like to work with them. Listen to their ideas. Always let them see that you believe their work is important and that you respect them.

- Do not work with only one healer. Always have several work with you. The risk in working with only one is that he or she may be a quack who is interested only in power and fame. Even a healer who is genuine may become too proud and take risks to get more glory. Also the other healers will probably become jealous and may try to give your chosen healer a bad reputation among the people.

  Several healers working together as a group can watch each other's activities. If one of them tries to do things that may harm the group's reputation, the others will probably prevent it.

- Always insist that the healers fulfil their role responsibly. This means not only caring for people in the best way. The healers must also give others — especially doctors and nurses — a good image of their medicine and of themselves. Because of this they should not take risks in treating people who are very sick or dangerously ill. Explain to the healers that it is better to send people who are extremely ill to the medical doctors if possible. Say that if a person dies in a hospital people will think that the death resulted from the illness. But if the person was treated by traditional healers, medical doctors may say that the healers caused the death. Stress that this would harm their reputation.

How to deal with quacks and dangerous traditional practices

If you notice that a healer is doing dangerous things that could cause harm, try first to find out whether these are genuine traditional practices or just a personal method used by a quack. Ask other healers what they think of these practices. Do they use them themselves? If not, why do they not use them? Ask them also whether these practices are widely used by other healers. This will help you to know whether these practices are just the work of a quack or whether they are common features of traditional healing.

Quacks

Genuine traditional healers will not defend or support quacks, especially if you stress that quacks damage the reputation of all good healers and of traditional medicine. Decide with them what can be done to oblige the quacks to stop their bad and dangerous practices. The good healers may not know what to do but at least they will understand that you want to protect them and their medicine by opposing the quacks.

Speak about the problem with the camp's leaders and authorities. You may find that even the leaders are worried about taking action although they may understand that quacks do dangerous things that should be stopped. People are often afraid of quacks because they claim to have magic powers. They do not want to turn the quacks into their enemies. They are afraid that the quacks will seek revenge and make them become sick or even die.

Tell officials from the organizations in charge of protecting the refugees or the displaced populations (UNHCR or the International Committee of the Red Cross, for example). They should do what is necessary if people's safety is at risk.

Controversial or dangerous traditional practices

Sometimes a treatment that is widely practised by healers, and not only by quacks, may be controversial or dangerous. Discuss such treatments with senior health workers or camp administrators if possible. Examples of treatments that could be dangerous are burning or cutting the skin, and wrapping babies with a high fever in warm blankets and extra clothes.

Another thing to remember about traditional healing is its cost. People who go to healers may be desperate for help, either for themselves or for a member of their family. They may be prepared to pay almost anything for help. Some healers, and especially quacks, may take advantage of this and demand large amounts of money for their services. Before you agree to work with a traditional healer, get some idea of how much they charge their clients.

Traditional medicine and the mentally ill

Some kinds of mental illness are very obvious. People with these illnesses may be agitated, afraid, talk nonsense or hear voices that do not exist. They may laugh and sing a lot and sleep very little.

Sometimes the mental illness is depression. Persons who are depressed are very sad, think that they have no value, have no hope and may want to kill themselves. These symptoms sometimes disappear without treatment within a few months. They may also continue for much longer and there is always a risk that a depressed person may commit suicide. Even after long periods of recovery, people may become depressed again. This is described in more detail in Unit 4, page 42.

It is doubtful whether persons such as these — with psychoses like schizophrenia or severe depression — can be cured by traditional healers. However, if healers are good people who treat those who seek their help kindly and humanely, there is no reason to worry. Let them try. They may be able to help those who come to them, even if they cannot cure them. After all, some mental illnesses go away without any treatment. Traditional healers may have a positive effect on a person's mental health. Still, for most people with mental illness, it is best to treat them with medical drugs as well as giving them traditional treatment. People treated by both healers and scientific medicine are more likely to make a good recovery than people who receive only the medical drugs. Remember to check carefully that the traditional treatment is acceptable and does not make people suffer or frighten them.

Most traditional healers admit that they cannot treat people with mental illnesses but some claim that they can. Be careful. It is most likely that the healers who claim this are honest and good people who believe that they have healed people who recovered by themselves. But they could also be quacks who use dangerous treatments.

Traditional treatment for the mentally ill

Physical treatment

Physical treatment usually consists of frightening and painful experiences. People may be severely beaten, burned in various places all over the body or forced to drink disgusting things. They may be badly frightened because they are made to think they will die or be killed.

The purpose of this kind of traditional treatment is to produce a shock which is supposed to bring the person back to reality. But, in fact, the person may get worse. Sometimes a person may seem to get better but the improvement does not last. Severe pain can reduce psychological suffering for a short time but it does not remove it. Those who use these methods claim success by showing temporary improvement but the person gets worse afterwards.

It is important to remember:

- Such methods are not treatment. They are forms of torture inflicted on people who are mentally ill.

- These methods cannot cure the mentally ill. Their condition is likely to become worse.

- These methods are not ethical. No one has the right to impose needless suffering on people who cannot defend themselves.

- Report use of these methods to the authorities and the organizations responsible for refugees and displaced populations. They should act to stop these practices.

Magic healing methods

Magic cures are performed through rituals that are different in each culture. In some places only the healer and the person who is mentally ill, and possibly the family, are involved in the rituals. In other places a large crowd may take part.

Magical treatment takes different forms. Special offerings might be made to a spirit that is thought to be seeking revenge because the sick person has offended it. Or an evil spirit that is thought to have possessed the person through black magic may be driven out. In some cultures a lost soul may be searched for.

The religious beliefs of some relief workers prevent them from accepting magical practices that they believe are witchcraft and the worshipping of false gods. These workers may oppose magic healing methods. Magic cures usually do not harm and may help people. There is no medical reason to oppose them.

These cures can be particularly helpful if the healers ask the spirit that is thought to possess a person to speak. It is believed that the spirit speaks through the mouth of the person. In this way problems can be spoken about easily. Normally the person would feel too ashamed to speak in this way of personal matters. Since it is thought that it is the spirit and not the person who is speaking, things can be said more easily. This can have a healing effect.

Sometimes persons who claim magical powers sprinkle special "lustral" water on people who are ill. Lustral water is prepared by reciting prayers, mantras or magic formulae over a container full of water. Often people treated with lustral water claim that they feel more relaxed and more comfortable and that their mind is clearer. Some say that they suffer less pain after this treatment. Healers may also blow on the head or on other parts of the body while saying prayers or magic words. This can also help some people calm down and feel less anxious.

Many other magic healing methods are medically acceptable if they are not associated with violent or painful practices.

Counselling

Traditional healers are usually old and wise and know how to listen and talk to people. They may give valuable advice, make useful comments or give explanations. This can reduce or take away people's guilt, worries and other painful feelings, such as the feelings we experience after a death or after other hurtful events.

Sometimes people find themselves in a very confusing and puzzling situation, such as during family conflicts. Healers can help people understand and sort out these situations. People trust healers and confide in them, so they find it easier to speak to healers and respect their advice.

Do not hesitate to involve traditional healers in counselling people who need to understand more clearly what their problems are. You may be able to involve some healers in group support work with people who have problems. It is often good to have both male and female traditional practitioners. You can involve traditional birth attendants as well as healers. Let each of them speak and listen. Say what you want to say, but do not take the leading role. Do not try to speed things up. People may need time to express their real problems.

Medication

Traditional healers prepare remedies for many kinds of physical complaint, such as headache, dizziness, fatigue, poor appetite and pain. These remedies can help people with these complaints. The complaints may be due to a physical illness but often they may have a psychological origin.

Some powerful medical drugs that are used for severe physical illnesses are made from substances that were first discovered in plants used by traditional healers. Examples are quinine (for malaria), digitalis (for heart failure), aspirin and rauwolfia (for high blood pressure, and for calming and sedating people).

Are there traditional remedies for severe mental illnesses? Are there plants that can cure people who hear voices, or who have delusions or speak nonsense? The answer is probably no.

Certain substances extracted from plants, such as mescaline, affect the mind. Healthy people who take these substances have hallucinations (they hear and see things that do not exist) and may become very anxious. These substances are dangerous and must not be used to treat the mentally ill.

Opium poppies and coca are plants with very powerful effects on severe pain and tiredness but they should not be used to treat mental illnesses. They can be dangerous because people quickly become dependent on them and cannot stop taking them.

Be careful if some healers say that they have plants to treat mental illness. Plants that act strongly on the mind are dangerous and may do more harm than good. Sometimes healers use cannabis (also called marijuana, hashish or ganja) but it should not be used as a medication. Many countries prohibit its use by law.

If a traditional healer claims to have a remedy for mental illness, ask what happens after the patient has taken this medicine. Ask what else the healer will do while the person is under the influence of the drug. Has anyone died during this treatment? Treatments that could put someone's life in danger or make people suffer are not acceptable.

Traditional remedies can be helpful and give good results, but be very careful with traditional remedies that are claimed to cure mental illness. They are probably useless and could be dangerous. Ask the advice of a scientifically trained medical doctor before you agree to healers using these remedies. If some families insist that remedies like this should be used, suggest that the treatment be supervised by a qualified health worker.

Complementary approaches

Traditional practitioners can provide useful services in health care, including mental health care. Acknowledge and praise their useful and safe skills, but do not believe that they can deal with all health problems. Like medical doctors, they cannot do everything. They can, however, help and heal many people with psychological problems and in painful and complicated circumstances.

It is less likely that traditional healers have the means of treating severe mental conditions, whereas medical doctors do have effective drugs.

The traditional and scientific approaches complement each other. Used together in the treatment of mentally ill refugees, they give better results than if just one approach is used.

Establish with healers a relationship based on mutual esteem, trust, respect and understanding. Support their practice and work with them as closely as possible. Remember, however, that quacks can do great harm, especially to those with severe mental disorders who cannot defend themselves. Quacks are not genuine traditional healers and they discredit traditional medicine.

Notes for camp administrators

Traditional medical practices are not dangerous just because they may seem odd, unfamiliar or shocking to the outsider. Before deciding that a traditional practice is dangerous, carefully observe what the healers are doing. Judge what they do from two standpoints — medical and ethical (moral).

Here are two examples of traditional practices. The first concerns superficial burns used as a treatment. The second is the habit of wrapping babies with high fever in warm clothes and blankets.

Example 1: Superficial burns

Some healers may make small superficial burns on certain parts of the body. Sometimes they do this together with acupuncture and call it "moxibustion", but sometimes it has no relation to Chinese medicine.

To decide whether this kind of treatment is acceptable, consider the following:

- How many burns are made, how big are they and where are they made? Are they superficial or deep? A few surface burns on parts of the body normally covered by clothes may be acceptable. Many deep burns, all over the body, are not acceptable. They are torture rather than treatment.

- What substances do the healers put on the burns? If it is earth or dung or any other dirty substance, it will cause infection and possibly death from tetanus. This is not acceptable, even on superficial burns.

- Is the treatment freely accepted by the person? In some societies, people do not mind scars. In other societies, scars are thought of as a bad thing. This is why burns on the face, neck or hands are probably bad and should be discouraged.

If you find a treatment not acceptable, you should have good reasons. Explain these reasons to the healers. Insist that they need to protect their reputation. They should never do anything that may give them a bad name.

Example 2: High fever and the risk of convulsions

When a baby has a high fever there is a risk that it will have convulsions. Severe convulsions or convulsions that happen again and again may seriously damage the brain. At the first convulsion, or preferably as soon as the baby's temperature rises above 39 °C, it is essential to cool the baby's body quickly. This can be done by bathing the baby in cold water and then placing it naked in a cool place or in a place where there is plenty of air. Medical doctors tell parents to do this because they know that the brain can be severely damaged during convulsions. Traditionally, however, people often do the opposite. They cover the baby with warm clothes and blankets. This dangerous tradition is very hard to stop.

Tell the healers that the baby may die from the disease that causes the fever whether the baby is covered or not covered and whether the fever is kept high or brought down. Ask the healers whether they have noticed that babies with high fever often have convulsions. They will tell you that they have. Ask them how they explain this. Then tell them how you explain it — by the effect of the temperature on the baby's brain. This does not happen when children are older because their brain is stronger. Ask them whether they have noticed that children who had severe convulsions when they were babies sometimes are normal afterwards but often are not normal. These children may not be bright or intelligent and may still have seizures.

Ask the healers how they explain this. Then tell them how you explain it — that it is because the baby's brain has been damaged during the convulsions. This is why we must try to prevent babies from having convulsions when their temperature is high.

Remember

- People do not change their habits or beliefs from one day to the next.

- Do not blame people for their traditions. They follow tradition because they believe it is right for their children, not because they are stupid or stubborn.

- People are more likely to follow your advice when they trust you. That is why it is important to build up a good relationship with them.

- Do not be surprised if people trust their traditional healers more than they trust you. Even if the healers are wrong to advise that a baby with high fever should be covered and you are right to advise the opposite, families are more likely to trust the healers than to trust you. That is why you need to get the healers on your side.

- Do not openly oppose the healers, even if they ask people to do something which you know is harmful. Stay calm and polite. Discuss with them, listen to their reasons and explain to them why medical doctors have a different opinion.

- The healers will trust you if you trust them. They will respect your opinion if you respect them. If you can convince them that what you suggest is right, they will be able to persuade the families to follow your advice.

Alcohol and other drug problems

Learning objectives

After studying this unit you should be able to:

1. Explain to key members of the refugee group, and to other relief workers, the risks of alcohol and other drug problems that refugees face.

2. Organize the refugee community to watch out constantly for this kind of problem in order to prevent or counter it.

3. Recognize people who already have problems related to alcohol and other drugs, or who are at high risk of developing such problems.

4. Arrange for suitable help for these people. Whenever possible this help should come from within the refugee community itself.

5. Establish links with health care services for referral of people who have taken a dangerous amount of alcohol or drugs. You should also be able to refer people with other complications that cannot be dealt with within the refugee community.

Alcohol and other drug problems are common in many societies. They may be lessened when people become refugees but they may also become worse.

There are several reasons for an increase in the risk of serious alcohol and other drug problems among refugees. Once the refugees themselves, as well as the authorities, are aware of why such risks occur, much can be done to prevent them and to help those who are affected.

How alcohol and other drug problems can occur

People who use alcohol or other drugs risk developing many problems. These include health, family and personal problems. As people use these substances more, they are more at risk. Some of the people you care for may have had these problems before they became refugees.

When people who use a lot of alcohol or drugs (heavy users) become refugees they may reduce or stop their use in the upset and confusion of their flight. But they are at serious risk of even more severe problems if nothing is done to prevent alcohol and drugs from becoming available to them. Those who used a lot before becoming refugees are most at risk once they have settled in the new community. A refugee community also has a potentially large number of new users, who could quickly become heavy users.

Some refugees may begin to use alcohol or other drugs as a way to avoid facing their real problems. Others may have a lot of time with nothing useful to do. The refugee may feel, "I don't care about the future or what happens to me or to other people." When families and society stop controlling people's behaviour in the normal way, young people in particular may start taking alcohol or drugs.

For alcohol and other drug problems to appear, suppliers must find a market among the refugees. If the refugees can pay for drugs, the drugs will soon be supplied. Suppliers of drugs (drug dealers) can easily take advantage of refugees and use them for their own purposes. They may use the refugees for illegal activities and pay them with alcohol or other drugs. They may look for ways of supplying the refugees without the knowledge of the authorities.

Refugees risk a lot by taking alcohol or other drugs regularly. These substances can seriously damage health, and when people are living in poor conditions the damage to health is even greater. When refugees spend the small amount of money they have on drugs, they make life even more difficult for others. Social problems caused by drug use can affect not only the family but also the refugee community as a whole.

If refugees use alcohol and other drugs regularly, they will make little effort to improve their living conditions. This affects all the refugees. Even if a few people begin to drink a lot or take other drugs, it affects the confidence and discipline of the whole community.

What you can do

Help the refugees to organize themselves to prevent a demand for alcohol and drugs within their community. It is also important to prevent outsiders from supplying the refugees with drugs.

Helping the community

You may need to tell the leaders of the refugee community about the risk of people starting to use alcohol or other drugs. Warn them that outsiders may try to create a demand for alcohol and other drugs.

Community leaders should understand that refugees are an easy target for drug dealers. This is especially true if the refugees are not well organized as a community and have little or no hope of returning to a normal social life again.

Encourage the community leaders to watch out for problems. Ask if they think that the use of alcohol and other drugs has already begun or is increasing. Do they think these problems could soon appear? If so, they could ask individual refugees or groups for help in preventing the problems before they begin. They could try to get the whole refugee community to act to prevent drug and alcohol use. They may be able to find out whether outsiders are trying to create a market. They could find out who these outsiders are and where they come from. Then they could decide on the best way to stop them.

Once the refugees and their leaders are aware of the risk, continue to discuss with them how to persuade people not to use drugs. Make everyone aware of how harmful the drug trade is. Persuade the refugees to take action to protect each other from starting or continuing to take drugs. Make it difficult for outsiders to profit from the conditions in which the refugees are living.

To prevent drug problems, everything should be done to improve and keep up the general welfare and morale of the refugees. All refugees should feel useful and should want to do their best for one another and for the whole community. If they have useful things to do and have some hope for the future, they will be less likely to take drugs. Warn the whole community that refugees who take drugs have more problems than people living in normal communities who take drugs.

Remember

- Stress the possible effects of drug use on the whole community.

- Help the community to understand the risks of alcohol and other drugs.

- Encourage the community always to keep watch for the beginnings of drug use.

- Arrange from time to time for the refugee community to commit itself publicly to stopping the use of alcohol and other drugs. The refugees must also commit themselves to stopping the illicit production and trade of alcohol and other drugs.

- Involve the whole community in group activities to help each other while they wait for a more permanent solution to their problem.

- Arrange for the refugees to discuss how they should organize themselves to prevent alcohol and other drugs from being used in their community.

- Always try to raise and maintain the refugees' hope.

By preventing the problems linked with the use of alcohol and other drugs you can prevent further harm to the refugees. Help them to understand this. They can then organize themselves to protect one another and the whole community from these problems.

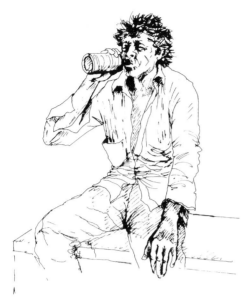

Some refugees will need special attention because of their alcohol use

Helping individuals

Some individual refugees will need special attention and help.

- Ask who uses alcohol or other drugs now and has problems because of this.

- Look out for behaviour that suggests alcohol or other drugs are being used. Also look for other signs and results of alcohol and drug use such as physical illness, injuries, drunkenness or strange behaviour.

- Find out which of the refugees are known to have been regular or heavy users of alcohol or other drugs before they became refugees. Such people are at special risk. Any demand or market for drugs is likely to start with them.

Previous heavy users or problem users

The refugees will usually know whether anyone in their community is using drugs in a harmful way. If there are no serious problems now, ask community leaders or others with influence if they know of people who were having problems from the use of alcohol and other drugs, or who used drugs every day, before they became refugees.

These persons are at special risk if alcohol or other drugs become available. Even if these persons are not using drugs now, the refugee leaders should try to involve them in community activities or meetings. This will help make them feel valued members of the group. It is important to give them a chance to do even small things for the welfare of all the refugees. Even as a refugee, the former drug taker should be helped to feel more valued than when he or she took drugs.

Current users

- The community usually knows who is taking alcohol or drugs. People may be seen doing this or may show signs of using alcohol or other drugs. Different drugs create similar problems, but remember that each drug has its own particular effect on users.

- Different kinds of drug may be used in different areas. Most people will know which drugs are commonly abused in their area. Learn to recognize the special features of withdrawal from drugs and dependence on drugs that are common in your area. You can recognize dependence on a particular drug by its effects and withdrawal symptoms.

- Some users may be taking alcohol or some other drug every day because they cannot cope without. These people are "dependent". Usually they have many problems. They damage their own health, they neglect their families, and they become a burden to their families and to the refugee community.

  People who are dependent on a drug need to take the drug regularly. If they do not have their drug, or if the drug is taken away from them, they suffer distress and withdrawal symptoms — a mixture of physical and mental symptoms. They feel better almost as soon as they take their drug again.

- Some drugs cause dependence more easily than others. Different drugs cause different kinds of withdrawal symptoms. Sometimes these symptoms seem to be mental — someone might have a strong desire for the drug, get angry easily and not be able to concentrate. Cocaine and cannabis cause this kind of withdrawal symptoms. Heroin and alcohol produce physical withdrawal symptoms. Withdrawal from heroin produces aches and pains all over the body. The person has difficulty sleeping, has a runny nose, watery eyes and sometimes gets diarrhoea. Someone who stops taking alcohol sleeps badly, becomes angry and restless easily, feels sick and may shake. In bad cases, the person may not be fully conscious. He or she may feel terrified, may see imaginary things and may even have fits like the fits that people with epilepsy sometimes have. Suddenly taking away alcohol from a person who is dependent on it can be dangerous. It can even cause death.

- Even people who are not dependent on drugs may have drug-related problems. These include health problems, poor nutrition, family problems, accidents, fights and other social problems. In a refugee camp, the use of drugs can lead to problems more quickly than in normal life.

- When illegal drugs are used, special problems occur. The distribution and sale of these drugs are unlawful and their suppliers are criminals. This brings special problems to the refugee community. The users of illegal drugs may also be considered criminals and so they may face extra risks.

- People who take drugs sometimes take an overdose (a dangerously large dose) or have a bad reaction to a drug. Some people have unusual reactions to drugs, but this is not common. Overdose occurs mostly with alcohol and medical drugs like barbiturates or tranquillizers. Overdose may lead to coma and even death.

Helping people who admit they have a drug problem

Sometimes drug users can be motivated to help themselves or accept the help of others. They can decide not only to stop taking drugs but also to live a more meaningful life. When drug users admit they have a problem they start to have a good chance of giving up the drug. Work patiently with such people to help them control their drug problems, stop using the drug and change all the behaviour that goes with drug use. This may be easier in a refugee camp than in normal life because, living with the other refugees, the drug user is less isolated.

- Find out who among the refugees is willing to help drug users. Organize a group of helpers and arrange for them to meet together. Explain to them the risks of heavy use of drugs. Discuss with them ways in which they can help users of drugs to control their problem.

- Explain that the most useful skill is the ability to talk to drug users in a friendly way. Suggest that each helper talks to one drug user as part of the community effort to control the problem. Tell them not to give orders. They should try to find out what the drug users feel about their problem and how likely it is that they can control it. Each helper should talk and listen to the drug user they are helping every day for a week. Then have another meeting with the helpers. At this meeting, they can tell one another about their experiences. They should describe their difficulties and discuss ways of overcoming them.

- Ask the helpers to discuss why drug users fail to control their problem. Explain that there may be many reasons for this. Drug users may not wish to change because they are not interested in any other aspect of life. They may be used to this way of life. They may not have any other interests. They may not feel part of society or of their families. They may have had unpleasant symptoms when they stopped using the drug for a time in the past.

- Ask the helpers what they can do to overcome these barriers.

- Suggest that the helpers continue to see the individuals they are helping regularly during the following weeks.

People can and do stop taking drugs, especially when others show an interest in helping them. The helpers, just by meeting drug users regularly, may help them to change. Change may also happen because the community shows an interest in the drug users. People who live in a refugee community can feel a particularly strong interest in others and sense of community care.

Fear of withdrawal symptoms can be a reason for not stopping drug use. Most users can stop taking their drug if they are determined to do so, without using any other drug. Sometimes stopping a drug suddenly can cause serious symptoms, and it is necessary to prescribe some medicine. Withdrawal is a threat to life only for the few people who are severely dependent on alcohol or drugs.

Helpers must know when special help is needed. It may not be easy to find a doctor in an emergency or when there is special problem. You or the helpers may have to handle the situation.

When possible, a link with the health care services should be set up for the times when you need to send people with severe complications to a specialist doctor. When doctors or nurses visit the refugee group, discuss the possibility of setting up this kind of link.

Problems that may arise when alcohol and other drugs are used

Drunken behaviour

One problem is drunken or intoxicated behaviour. A drunken person may be violent and aggressive. Some people are always aggressive after drinking alcohol, but they can usually control aggressive behaviour if they know that other people will not accept it. When a drunken person behaves violently in public it is best to take the person away or persuade the other people to go away. Never challenge someone who is drunk and aggressive or try to stop the behaviour. He or she may try to attack you. It is usually much better to agree with the drunken person and to try to get the person away from the situation that is causing the violent reaction.

Overdose

An overdose may cause a person to become unconscious. Watch an unconscious person carefully to avoid other harm. Pay special attention to the person's breathing. Patients who are unconscious after taking alcohol often have low levels of glucose in their blood. This can damage the brain, and the damage can remain even after the alcohol has been cleared from the body. An unconscious person should not be given anything by mouth; he or she may need to be given glucose by injection. A trained health worker should do this.

Withdrawal

The symptoms that people experience when they stop taking alcohol or other drugs can be relieved in various ways. Sometimes medicines may be necessary. Diazepam and similar medicines can help to prevent the dangerous withdrawal effects that occur with severe alcohol dependence. They should be given only for a short time and the dose should be reduced gradually.

People who stop taking alcohol may have times when they are not fully conscious. These people may have fits, or be confused. They may also see things that are not there. In such cases medicines such as diazepam may be given for a short time, and the doses gradually reduced.

People going through withdrawal from alcohol or other drugs should not be left alone. Someone they know well should stay with them. This should be someone who is able to communicate clearly with them and stimulate them to remain conscious. The surroundings should also be stimulating, with good light, for example. If the condition of the person going through alcohol withdrawal becomes much worse, a small amount of alcohol may be given, especially if there are no medicines available.

The helpers should also speak to the families of the alcohol and drug users they are helping. A person who cuts down or stops using drugs should be praised and congratulated on the achievement. Family, friends and helpers should show their satisfaction and give encouragement.

Helpers can tell drug users other things they can do to gain respect. Bring together the helpers and those who have stopped taking drugs to discuss how much others in the community appreciate the change. Helpers and former users can plan together things the former drug users can do that the community would value. They can discuss together how to avoid falling back into drug use.

Former drug users can plan ways to stop the supply of alcohol and other drugs to the refugees. In this way they will be helping the whole community and strengthening their loyalty to one another. They will have a sense of a united effort to protect themselves from being used by outsiders.

Helpers should keep in regular contact with the former users to help them to maintain the changes they have made in their lives. In this way they can also reach current drug users.

Helpers should encourage former drug users to speak to current users and help them stop using drugs. Explain to the helpers that regular contact over a long period is needed to make sure that former drug users do not start taking drugs again.

One way of helping people who have stopped taking alcohol or other drugs is to find them a useful task or encourage them to find a useful task. This task could be to help other drug users to stop taking drugs. Or it may be to stop the supply of drugs to the refugee community.

Everyone should show how much they value the efforts of the helpers. But remember that success depends greatly on the continuing organized efforts of the refugee community to prevent more drug problems occurring in future.

UNIT 8

Helping victims of torture and other violence

Learning objectives

After studying this unit you should be able to:

1. Recognize the problems and symptoms that may occur in other people who have been tortured or who have suffered other forms of violence.

2. Recognize the effects that torture or other abuse may have had on you. Learn how to deal with the memories of these painful experiences so that you will find it easier to help others.

3. Organize groups with other refugee workers to discuss your experiences in helping people who have been tortured and your feelings while helping these people.

4. Help these people through individual or group support.

Torture takes place in about one-third of countries. Torture means the infliction of physical or emotional pain, anguish, agony and torment in order to obtain information or to change the views of the tortured person. Torture methods are designed to force the victim to do what the torturer wants. Physical techniques include all kinds of beating and electric shock. People may also be deprived of food, water, sound or light, or submerged in water. Or they may be tortured with other kinds of violence and physical and sexual abuse. Psychological techniques such as false accusations, threats of death or fake executions are used to confuse the victim and break down resistance. The most common consequences are psychological ones such as fear, depression and nervousness. The person who has been tortured may experience difficulty in concentrating, may be unable to sleep or may have nightmares. These problems usually start immediately but in some cases they may begin months or years after the original torture. They may last for a long time.

Many refugees have also suffered other forms of violence, which may have been as severe as torture. They may have lost one or more family members and may even have witnessed their death. Some may have been wounded or physically disabled. They may have seen others starve or may have been bombarded during their escape.

How to recognize people who have been subjected to severe forms of violence

Everyone who suffers painful and very hurtful experiences reacts physically and emotionally in a similar way. They are not sick or weak. Usually they will get better with time. Here are some common reactions to severe violence:

- Some people think about the painful experience all the time. Some may even feel as if they are undergoing the same experience again and again. They may see vividly the violent event or torture.

- Some people feel sick and experience pain. This may lead them to visit a health worker more often than in the past. (See Unit 3.)

- Some have difficulties with sleep; they may be unable to fall asleep or they may wake up very early. (See Unit 2.)

- Some have bad dreams and nightmares.

- There may be loss of interest in life, loss of energy and a feeling of tiredness all the time. This can lead to difficulties with work or with daily tasks.

- Some people have problems with eating; they may eat too little or too much.

- Some lose interest in sex.

- Some have poor concentration, poor memory or tell the same story again and again.

- There may be a tendency to become angry about little things or change moods quickly.

- Some people feel afraid, nervous or jumpy.

- Some feel guilty about being alive when others have died.

- Some show no interest in other people or in their families.

- Some people avoid situations or discussions that remind them of the painful experience.

- Some drink too much alcohol or take drugs. (See Unit 7.)

Most people who have been tortured or treated violently show some of these symptoms. Someone who has suffered severe violence or torture may have most of these reactions. Every person is different and some people can tolerate suffering better than others, but any person who complains about several of these reactions will probably need extra support. This unit will help you to help these people.

How to recognize in yourself the effects of having been treated violently

Many refugees have gone through similar difficulties. Maybe you are a community health worker, a religious leader or a local healer and you realize that you have suffered the same kind of violence as the people around you. Because of this, you may even find it hard to listen to other people who want to talk about their problems.

People may expect that they can come to you for help at any time. Maybe you share this view. Perhaps you have been in this position in your community for many years. Of course, your own life may have changed because of the trouble or the disaster that made you flee your homeland.

To find out whether you also need support, ask yourself some questions about your past since you left your home.

- Have you had an opportunity to talk to others about your experiences?

- Do you have such an opportunity now?

- Are you able to recall what happened to you and your family without crying or getting angry?

- Do you ever have a chance to relax after long days of work?

- Can you be pleasant and nice with the people you work with and with family members?

If your answer to most of these questions in "No", you may have had a difficult time. This will make it hard to support others who have lived through similar hardships.

To find out if supporting others will be difficult for you, ask yourself some further questions:

- Do people seem too ill-at-ease in your presence to talk about the violence or the torture they have endured?

- When people discuss their experiences with you, do you find it hard to give them your full attention?

- Do your thoughts often wander and you feel as though you are not really there?

- Do you get very bored, tired, annoyed or restless?

If your answer to most of these questions is "Yes", it may be wise to organize some kind of support for yourself.

How to help yourself and others to recover from violent experiences

If you want to support others, it is best to solve your own problems first. When you have dealt with your own hardships you will be better able to support others. This section explains how to set up a support group for yourself and other refugee workers in your camp or area. You can use such a group to support other refugees who have suffered torture or other kinds of violence. This section also explains how to counsel individuals.

In some situations almost everyone has experienced violence or torture. This can be the case, for example, after a war. In these situations a group approach may be the best way of helping people. You can still give special attention to individuals who had an experience that was not shared by many others, or who have taken part in group sessions but still continue to have serious symptoms.

How to set up a support group for colleagues

Invite some colleagues to form a mutual support group to exchange experiences in dealing with victims of violence. If your culture permits, the group should include both men and women because they often deal with their problems in different ways. The members of the group can come from different professions or backgrounds. Your group might include a nurse, a local healer, a local chief or a religious leader, a doctor, or a teacher, for example. A good size for a group is between 6 and 10 people.

When the group first meets, the members should know clearly their reasons for coming together. These may include:

- To give one another the opportunity to talk about the past.

- To gain experience on how to deal in a group with the effects of torture and other forms of violence. Later each member can start a separate group to help other victims of violence.

- To learn from one another's experiences about effective ways of helping people who have suffered.

- To allow group members to talk about their feelings in dealing with victims.

- To learn to respect confidentiality. What you tell each other must remain within the group. Also respect confidentiality when supporting other people later.

In the first or second session the group members can discuss how the group should be organized and how its meetings can best be fitted into the local routine. For example, meetings may be held weekly and last between 1 and $1\frac{1}{2}$ hours. Group members can take turns in leading the meeting.

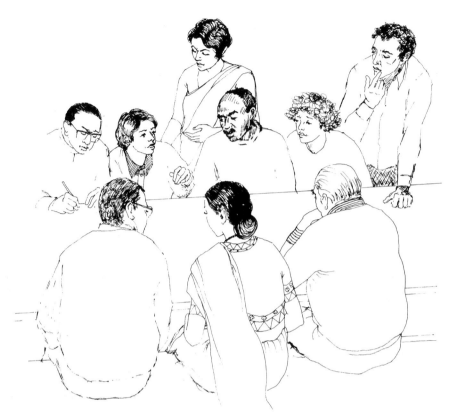

Invite some colleagues to a mutual support group to exchange experiences in dealing with victims of violence

Once you know one another a little better, spend one meeting on group relaxation exercises (see Unit 2). Each subsequent meeting should start with these group relaxation exercises.

At the next two or three meetings discuss stress and people's reactions to stress. The following text may be helpful. With the other group members you can adapt this text to your circumstances and then make copies of it. Later the copies can be used for group and individual counselling.

Text to use in counselling victims of violence or torture

What has happened to you is so terrible that anyone with the same experience would have the same complaints. Most people who undergo extreme stress, for example, in an accident, war or rape, react automatically. Usually they react very well and do what is necessary to escape or to survive. When the danger is over they may feel shock and find it hard to believe that they have escaped. They may tremble and feel fear, anger or grief for hours or days. It is very

114

comforting to have someone to reassure you and tell you it is all over and that you are safe.

Then you start to go over the experience. Often you do not want to be reminded of what has happened. You go on living as you have always lived. Or you do not want other people to talk about the past. At other times it is as though all the terrible things are happening again. You remember everything, you see all the details before you, and you feel unhappy, afraid, humiliated or angry. Most people are worried about this process of not remembering anything and, then, remembering everything.

People may change. For example, a man may be irritable all the time although before he was always a likeable person. He may avoid contact with other people although before he liked to chat, play games or dance. Or he may drink too much or take drugs, which he never did before.

If you have been tortured, remember that torture is used to damage the person-ality. Torturers often try to frighten people by telling them that they will have difficulties with sleep or with sex. If you have been frightened like this, remember the words of the torturer. Under torture, victims can enter into a state of mind that later makes them think the threats may be real for the rest of their lives. Remember that the torture was not your fault. You do not have any responsibility for what happened during the torture.

The group sessions will help you to digest the painful memories little by little, just as you take your food in small pieces so that you can digest it more easily. It is normal to have problems like nightmares, painful memories, irritability and crying. Do not worry that you might be going crazy because you have never felt like this before.

Some people explain their hardship with ideas from their local culture. They may say that their problem is caused by witchcraft, or by the anger of spirits, or their Supreme Being. Or they may think that they have lost their soul, or that they are being punished for something they did either in this life or in a previous one. This way of looking at your problem will not help you.

Everyone experiences more or less the same problems after such hardships. Some people feel ashamed or guilty, perhaps because they were humiliated, perhaps because they imagine that they could have saved others, or even because they are still alive. Some people even feel like a traitor despite all the suffering they have been through. But most of them could not have done otherwise and they did the best they could in the situation. Some people were forced to do bad things in the past. In that case it is best to go through the proper ceremony or ritual to pray or to make a sacrifice in order to obtain forgiveness and prevent the anger of the spirits or the Supreme Being.

These sessions will help you to feel better in the future. Many people all over the world have found comfort and support in this way. Their memories of what happened have become less painful and less frequent. You will also be able to enjoy life again, even though at first it may only be from time to time. But to feel better, you will also have to go through some hard times. You will have to face the painful past before you can get rid of it.

From time to time you will still hear stories or see things that will remind you of the horrors you have gone through. But slowly you will begin to feel better. Think of your problem as an old wound with a lot of dirt in it. To heal the wound you have to take out the dirt. This may hurt a lot, but only then can the wound close and a scar form. Sometimes the scar still hurts. It can hurt by itself, or because the weather changes, or because somebody puts pressure on it. But the scar is also a good thing — it prevents more serious illness and it will protect you in the future.

At the next 10 meetings or so you can discuss each other's experiences with violence and how they have affected your lives. The group members can help one another to feel the emotions linked with the painful events. After 10–15 meetings the group members may want to continue the meetings until they feel that they have had enough opportunity to tell their own stories. Telling a story several times helps a person pick up the threads of life again. Make sure that sooner or later each member gets the opportunity to talk about the past.

During these meetings you can use the various techniques mentioned in the other chapters of this manual. As well as breathing and relaxation techniques or physical exercise, it is important to find some forms of recreation.

To help others, start similar groups with victims of violence. Run the groups along the lines of your colleague support group. Again, use the various techniques described in this manual. The colleague support group can continue to meet from time to time to provide help.

How to help individuals who have suffered serious violence

It has been explained above that it is better to use a group approach if you work in a situation where many people have had painful emotional experiences, such as after a war. Sometimes, however, an individual approach is better — for instance, if the victim's experience is not shared by many others or if the person has already been a member of a group but still has serious problems. Some people feel so frightened by group meetings that it may be good at least to start with individual counselling. For some people, their position in a community or political movement may make it impossible for them to talk in front of others about the violence or torture they suffered. It would be best to help them individually.

This section outlines a step-by-step approach to supporting individuals with serious problems. You will probably need between 10 and 15 sessions. However, psychological and social problems can be so complex that the person who seeks help may need more sessions. Each session will take 40–45 minutes. For the first three sessions ask the person to bring along one or more family members or friends.

This part of the unit is not simple. It would be a good idea at the beginning of each session to repeat to yourself what you are going to do in the session.

Plan for individual support sessions

Session 1

Goal: To create a relationship of trust and faith with the person needing help and with the family members or friends who have come with him or her.

At the first meeting try to make the person feel at ease.

Find a quiet place where other people will not interrupt you. Give your name and say what your job is. Make sure you have at least 45 minutes free to talk. Listen carefully with all your attention so that the victim of violence and possibly the family members can speak openly. Show respect. Treat the victim with dignity and understanding. Say that all you are told will be kept confidential. Show that you care about the person seeking help. Ask questions when you are not sure what the person means. Simple questions are best, such as "What happened then?" or "What did you feel like when that happened?" Help the person to express feelings or talk about the past by nodding your head, by saying "I understand" or by asking simple questions. It is very important that you let the person talk first, without trying to give advice or solve the problem.

First allow the person seeking help and his or her relatives to explain what happened. Let them tell the whole story. They should tell you what they did, what emotions they felt, what they felt physically and what they thought, especially at difficult moments. It may be useful to take a few notes, especially when people talk about their complaints and symptoms. When they have finished their stories, use the list of 14 common complaints on page 111 and note how many of those complaints are present.

To end this session, tell the person that you will meet together once a week another 10–15 times. Say that many people like to talk about what happened to them. Say that at the end of the sessions the person will still have problems and will still be preoccupied with the past. But he or she will be able to go on living and pick up the threads of life. Thank the other family members or friends for coming and tell them that they will also be given information and advice. Then make the next appointment.

If people seeking help have many social problems, first help them to sort out their problems and get their lives in order. This may take one or two extra sessions. You can help them individually to solve their problems by making a list of what they think are the most serious and the least serious problems. Help them to think of different ways to solve their problems and to decide on the best way to solve each one. Encourage them to take action and see how it works. Talk about the positive aspects of the action. In this way, those seeking help will learn to have more confidence both in themselves and in you. They will start to feel they have some control over their lives again.

Session 2

Goal: To enable the person seeking help to learn relaxation techniques.

Teach the relaxation exercises described in Unit 2, page 25. It may take several sessions for people to learn to do the exercises without your help. If there is a tape recorder available, they can listen to a tape of the relaxation exercise twice a day. After a week they should be able to do the daily exercise without the tape. Do the relaxation exercises at every session. If possible, the victim of violence should continue doing the exercises even after the series of sessions has finished. You can teach relaxation exercises to individuals or to groups.

If possible, also teach some simple massage techniques or encourage the use of massage techniques known in your culture (see page 27). This may be especially helpful when partners have trouble talking with each other or have difficulty with sexual relations. Explain to them that massage helps a person to relax and that it gives new strength to both body and soul.

Session 3

Goal: To provide information about stress and common responses to stress.

Explain what stress is and how people react to stress (see page 16). Read the text that you used at the meetings of the colleague support group. Give a copy of the text to the person you are helping or give a tape recording of the text if the person has a tape recorder or can borrow one. The person should either read or listen to the text repeatedly until he or she is able to repeat the important parts to a family member or friend.

Then ask the victim of violence and the family member or friend if they recognize in their own lives some of the things mentioned in the text. Take care that the partner gets an opportunity to express views about the problem. Ask whether the partner and other family members feel that this problem affects them (such as through violence at home) or affects their environment (such as through alcohol abuse). Thank the partner or friend for coming. At the end of the session, write down the problems mentioned by the family members or friend and the person who came for help.

Session 4

Goal: To identify the most frightening moments.

Let the victim of violence tell the whole story of what happened. Ask what the most difficult periods were. The answer may be "When the war started", or "When the drought came", or "When the soldiers started shooting", or "When they tortured me" or "When we had to leave our land". Most people will mention two or three difficult periods. Write down the answers.

Next, mention the first difficult period the person told you about. Ask whether during this period there were any especially difficult or agonizing moments. People may mention one moment or several moments. Write these moments down. They may be, for example, "When they blindfolded me", "When he took out his knife" or "When I heard the planes coming". Then for every one of those moments ask the following questions and write down the answers carefully:

- What did you do at that moment?

- What did you feel in your body?

- What else did you feel? (If the person does not answer, ask, "For example, did you feel afraid, or angry, or powerless, or ashamed?")

- What did you think?

- What did you hear?

People may become emotional in replying to these questions. This is good. It helps them to relive some of what happened. If a person hesitates do not hurry. Some people need time to talk, or to cry, or to be silent. After this pause, you may say that you understand that it can be difficult to find words for what has happened. Ask whether the person wants to carry on with the session.

Then take another difficult period that has been mentioned. Again ask about the most difficult moments. Write down the answers. For each moment, ask the same questions: "What did you do?", "What did you feel?", "What did you think?" and so on.

Then ask whether one particular period was more difficult than the others. Write down the periods in order of the most difficult, the second most difficult, and so on.

At the end of this session, express in your own words your appreciation of the person's courage in talking about these experiences.

Sessions 5–7

Goal: To change the effect of the violence or torture on the life of the person.

Tell the victim of violence that during these sessions both of you will go back to the painful periods mentioned in the previous sessions. It will not be easy, but being cured is like the healing of an abscess — it hurts to take the pus out but then one begins to feel better and the abscess disappears.

First explain that, if the experience of remembering becomes too painful, the person can take a pause. All the person has to do is lift one finger, or a hand. Demonstrate this by putting your hand in a resting position and raising your first finger a little, or raising your hand.

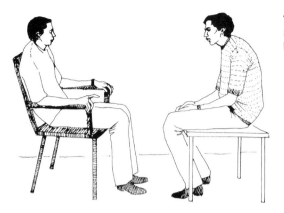

The refugee can use the finger signal to indicate he wants a pause

Ask the person you are helping to relax in the way learned earlier. Then go back to the least painful moment of the most difficult situation which you wrote down during the previous session. Help the victim to cast his or her mind back by reading the details that you wrote down about that moment. Use the present tense, as if it is happening now. From your notes talk through what the person does, feels, thinks, hears, smells and so on. For example, "Again you are in your cell. The footsteps are coming. You think, 'They are coming to fetch me to torture me.' You feel afraid. You feel them slap your face . . ."

If the person signals that he or she wishes to pause, say, "Let the images slowly go away until you don't see them any longer. Continue breathing and relaxing the way you have learned until you feel at ease." When the person is relaxed, take up the memory at the point where you stopped when the person gave the signal. After you have gone through the whole difficult situation again, ask the person to relax once more. Then repeat the process, talking through the difficult moment from beginning to end.

Again ask the person to relax. Ask whether the confrontation was less painful the second time than the first time. Then ask whether the person still felt tense as you repeated the episode. Say that it is better to repeat the exercise again until the tension feels less. Talk through the difficult moment again. Afterwards ask whether the tension is reduced or perhaps has almost gone. If the answer is "Yes", ask the person to repeat the following words: "It is all over and it is all finished. I can let go of it. I am free of it."

After you have gone all the way through this moment three or four times without the person having to stop you, take a more painful moment from that most difficult period and do the same thing. Keep doing this until you have gone through all the painful moments of that most difficult period. In one session you can go through one, two, three or four moments of one difficult period. After the session, tell the person that he or she has succeeded in completing the most difficult part of the healing process. Say that if he or she goes on like this, the counselling sessions will soon be completed.

Sessions 6 and 7

In the same way as in Session 5, confront the person with the other two or three difficult periods that you noted down in Session 4.

Session 8

Goal: To help the person to stop avoiding certain situations or other people.

Tell the person that you will have two or three more sessions together. Explain that in the future the person will sometimes feel disturbed again. Say that this is normal, like an old scar that has healed but sometimes hurts again.

In this session find out what other problems are troubling the person. Focus especially on things that the person would like to do but is afraid of doing. Write down the answers. If the person does not mention a problem, repeat the text used in Session 3. Read the text slowly. Ask the person seeking help to stop you when you mention something that is difficult. Again make a list of the problems mentioned. Then ask what is the least difficult and what is the most difficult problem. For instance, the least difficult problem may be to walk through the camp and the most difficult problem may be to leave the camp to work on a vegetable plot because it makes the person think of bombardments or mines.

First suggest an exercise to help with the least difficult problem. Start this first exercise during the session. Start by doing the relaxation exercise and then leave your counselling room or meeting place together. If the least difficult problem is to walk through the camp, walk together through the camp. Do this for at least 20 minutes. Then get the person to go through the relaxation exercise for at least 20 minutes before going home. The person must repeat the walk, followed by the relaxation exercise, every day. At first the person may do the walk with a partner or friend, but after one or two weeks it must be done alone. If the person agrees to try to do these things every day with a friend and eventually alone, make a new appointment for three weeks later.

Session 9

Take the next most difficult problem. Do the same exercise as in Session 8. The person seeking help should continue this again for another three weeks. If necessary, a further session can then be held to deal with a third problem.

The final session

Goal: To spot setbacks. To integrate the difficult, painful experience in the person's life and, if possible, find a meaning for it.

Explain that this is the last session. Express your appreciation for the way the person has been able to face up to the difficult past. Give assurance that the improvement will continue gradually and that setbacks will usually be over come without help from anyone. Recovery from setbacks usually takes a few hours or at most a few days. After that time anyone who still feels unable to carry on alone can make another appointment with you.

The victims of violence or family members may feel that some ceremonies, prayers or offerings are necessary. This may help them. They may want to join a group of people who have had similar experiences or who share a political goal. That would be a good thing to do. Remember, it is important for the person to find a useful role in life.

Tell victims of violence that people sometimes discover that suffering has had some positive effect, even though at that moment they may find it hard to believe.

Helping victims of rape and their communities

Learning objectives

After studying this unit you should be able to:

1. Describe the problem of rape among refugee women and girls.

2. Recognize and assist victims of rape.

3. Help the refugee community discuss the problem of rape and learn not to blame the victim.

4. Speak out on behalf of rape victims for better services and programmes.

Rape is a form of sexual violence commonly committed against refugee women and girls. It can occur in their home countries, during their flight, or in refugee camps when there is no protection. Sexually violent acts such as rape are very frightening experiences for female refugees. Some of those who are raped find the experience so traumatic that they commit suicide. Rape affects the life of the victim and her family as well as the community in which she lives.

Some facts about rape and rape trauma

- Rape is a violent and forceful act. It is commonly committed against refugee women and girls.

- Rape should not be considered primarily as a sexual act. Men who rape women and girls do so to gain control and to show power. They may be angry and want to hurt someone.

- Rape and other forms of sexual violence are against the human rights of refugee women and girls.

- Any refugee woman, of any age, may be raped. She may be over 60 years of age or younger than nine years.

- Refugee women and girls may be raped in their own countries, in camps in the first country they arrive in, or in the country where they finally resettle.

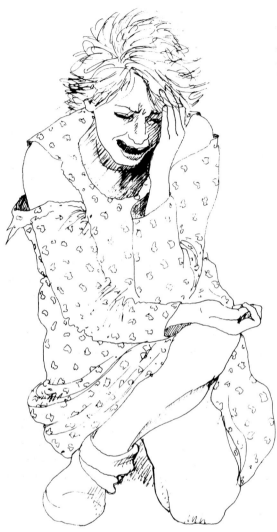

Rape should not be considered primarily as a sexual act. Men who rape women and girls do so to gain control and to show power

- Men who are supposed to protect refugee women and girls are sometimes those who rape them.

- The rape of refugee women and girls is often planned in advance.

- Rape has serious harmful effects on refugee women and girls. It can change their lives.

Rape takes place in all countries of the world, against females of every race and every social and economic class. Statistics show that every five minutes a woman is raped. Many women do not report rape. Rape is often not a means to

124

sexual satisfaction. Studies suggest that it is most often used as a way for men to show their power over women. This applies particularly to refugees, as after war men are more likely to feel the need to regain power and control. Rape is only one form of violence against women. Other forms include family or domestic violence.

Female refugees may be raped at any time during their flight. They may be raped by pirates, border guards, patrol-men, other refugees, and "cayottes" — men who are paid large sums of money to help refugees flee illegally to other countries. The cayottes may rape women and girls in exchange for safe passage. They may do this instead of, or often as well as, taking money. In refugee camps women may sometimes be forced to have sex with men in authority in exchange for food rations and other necessities.

Men can be raped too

Men can also be raped. Men and boys may find it difficult to admit that they have been raped. They may feel that they are weak because they were not able to stop the rape from happening. They may not know that many other men were also raped.

Make sure that men can talk to a male counsellor in private. If many men come forward you could set up a support group for male victims of rape.

How to recognize rape victims

Refugee women and girls are often discouraged by their culture or religion from revealing that they have been raped, or from openly discussing their experience. This means that the problem remains hidden. When the problem is kept secret, it is difficult to help the victim. Try to meet privately with the person you think may be a rape victim. If possible a female refugee worker should do this. If the woman or girl is ashamed or unwilling to discuss her problem, ask discreet and indirect questions.

Some ways to identify rape victims

- Study background materials and refugee stories describing the circumstances of the escape. This information will help you to identify situations where rape may have occurred.

- Look for signs of post-traumatic stress. These might be nightmares, loss of appetite, sadness, fear, confusion or isolation. Sometimes the rape victim will talk about suicide. (See Unit 8.)

- Look for signs of physical violence on the victim. Sometimes the husband or other male family members may physically assault a rape victim because they believe she is no longer clean.

- Meet with the family to find out whether they have noticed a problem.

- Keep close contact with community members and leaders to discover whether a young girl or woman is being kept in isolation or whether people talk about her in a disapproving way. This may indicate that she is a rape victim.

Unfortunately for the rape victim, when the other refugees in the camp learn of her experience they may speak ill of her. The relief worker should meet with elders, religious leaders and other community leaders to find out whether there are rumours and disapproving talk about a refugee woman or girl who has been raped.

Some reactions to rape

Depression is a common reaction to rape, but the rape victim may also experience some of the following emotions:

— feelings of shame and disgrace or of humiliation (loss of face in the community);

— guilt about having brought disgrace to the family;

— anger;

— a feeling of resignation to fate or destiny;

— constant thoughts about her problem;

— self-isolation or isolation by her family;

— fear of strangers;

— nightmares or inability to sleep;

— poor appetite;

— lack of hope about the future or fear of change;

— fear of the future;

— helplessness;

— feeling dirty and soiled.

How to help rape victims

- Respect confidentiality by keeping information private in all rape cases. Strict confidentiality is essential. If the rape victim feels that a counsellor or relief worker cannot be trusted, the victim will suffer and the relief worker will not be able to do the job properly. For example, relief workers should be very careful not to tell a story that a rape victim may think is her own story, even if they do not mention her name. The rape victim, and other women, may feel that the relief worker cannot be trusted to keep their experiences secret. This may discourage other victims who have not yet told anyone of their experience from coming forward.

Confidentiality means not telling other people the victim's name and not disclosing her identity. Written information or files on the victim must be kept locked away from others. Some rape victims may prefer not to tell their stories to the relief workers, or even to their husbands and families.

- Recognize that rape and other forms of sexual violence against refugee women and girls are common. Women and girls who have been raped may not wish to talk to other people about their tragedy because they feel they have become shameful.

- If the victim has contracted a sexually transmitted disease or is pregnant from rape, make sure that she attends a medical facility or health centre. Do not force her to make decisions but make it very clear to her that she needs professional medical help.

- Show your support and care for the rape victim. Listen to her stories. Do not make moral judgements about her.

- Allow the victim to talk when she is ready to do so. She will talk when she feels she can trust you. Do not push her into making decisions.

- Do not make the victim repeat her rape story many times.

- Find ways to end the social isolation of the rape victim.

- Discuss your feelings with other relief workers to share experiences.

- Organize support groups for rape victims and for yourself. Everyone needs someone to rely on for emotional and social support and understanding.

- Help the authorities to prepare leaflets or general written information in the languages of the refugees. Information should be available to everyone. Not only female refugees, but also men, will become better informed about rape and sexual violence in general.

Four steps to treatment

Once there is enough evidence that a young girl or woman who has experienced rape is suffering from its consequences, the following steps need to be taken to ensure that she receives attention and treatment:

Step 1. Explain to the rape victim that what happened is not her fault. This is especially important for those women who, because of religion or culture, believe that this tragedy happened to punish them for something bad they had done.

Step 2. After the rape the victim usually thinks that she is unclean and bad. In some cultures people feel that a woman's value lies in her virginity, modesty and female "cleanliness". In these cultures it is commonly believed that rape makes a woman less valuable and leaves her unclean. To help change such beliefs and attitudes, seek the help of religious leaders. For example, they could help the victim by performing special religious cleansing ceremonies and by praying for, and with, her and her community.

Step 3. Encourage the victim to express anger at the rapist. Blaming the rapist may stop her from blaming herself.

Step 4. Teach the victim some ways to avoid being raped in the future. After dark it is safer to go in groups rather than alone. Refugees should try to set up a system for reporting men who attempt rape to the proper authorities.

Very severe trauma

The trauma of the rape victim is sometimes so severe that its effects cannot be relieved in a short time even with emotional support and medication. Only continuous attention until the victim feels whole again will be successful.

Relief workers may discuss the following steps with a trained counsellor to agree on a more intensive approach to the victim with severe trauma:

Step 1. Ensure that the rape victim has access to a trained counsellor with whom she can meet for at least one hour a week.

Step 2. The counsellor should work in a team with a trained female health worker or welfare worker of the same culture as the rape victim.

Step 3. The counsellor and the refugee worker should work closely with other service providers, members of the community and religious leaders so that all learn to deal sympathetically and skilfully with rape victims.

Step 4. The refugee worker and service providers should cooperate to find useful activities for the rape victims. Most refugee women say that doing something that meets their own or their families' needs for survival keeps them from thinking all the time about the rape.

Men who have witnessed the rape of family members also suffer trauma. They need help to overcome this trauma.

Support groups

One way to help rape victims is to organize a support group. The members of the group meet together to support one another and help break down the isolation that each individual feels.

The group should be encouraged to meet frequently. Group activities should be things that the group members find interesting and worth while, and that occupy their minds with positive thoughts. This will prevent them from always thinking about their rape. They will feel reassured that they can still do useful and necessary things. Also, the support group will help each woman to stop feeling like a victim and to start feeling positive about herself and her contribution to the work of the group.

A support group could include both rape victims and women who have suffered in other ways but have not necessarily been raped. The group can discuss individual problems, but opening discussions should focus on the group's general needs rather than immediately dealing with rape or other forms of abuse. Once the group members feel at ease with each other, the group leader may introduce a general discussion about sexual violence against women.

The group should meet once a week if possible. Meetings should be both informative and interesting, so that the women will want to attend. The women themselves should agree on a convenient time and place for the group to meet. Meetings of the support group can also be used to train its members or improve their skills in activities such as sewing, reading and writing, women's health and nutrition, and ways of earning money.

Support group meetings should not be used for counselling or psychotherapy. Usually the relief worker will be able to learn, either directly or indirectly, about group members' medical or psychological needs. The relief worker can do this by listening to discussions during training and other activities. A variety of training models and exercises may be used in support group meetings.

Points to stress during treatment

1. Victims of rape and other forms of abuse are not responsible for the rape or abuse.
2. The victims are not alone. Many other women have overcome their abuse and are leading normal lives.

More suggestions for relief workers

You will often have to refer rape victims to health or welfare professionals for help. It is important that you know what resources exist in the camp and how to guide victims to the person who can help them. Some rape victims will need help from a trained counsellor to overcome their emotional problems. Do not try to provide intensive emotional counselling yourself. Your role should be:

— to help break the social isolation of the rape victim;

— to help the victim understand the problem;

— to help the victim stop blaming herself;

— to encourage the rape victim to become an active member of the women's community;

— to ensure that victims have access to services that meet their needs discreetly.

These five activities will help the victim gradually recover from the emotional and social scars of rape.

The rape victim may think of you as a member of her extended family. She may also see you as her only link with the outside world. Recognize this and maintain a warm and caring relationship with her.

Do not write notes about the rape victim in her presence. Refugees may believe that the information is going into their files and may prevent them from being resettled. Try to take notes as soon as the rape victim leaves. Do not rush her when she is meeting with you.

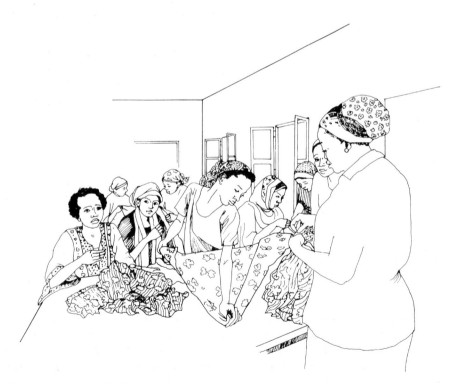

Help the rape victim become an active member of her community

Notes for camp administrators

Coordinating efforts to help rape victims

Relief workers and people providing services in the refugee camp should organize discussions of the problems of rape victims and of ways of improving services for them. One outcome of these discussions should be a list of steps to go through when working with rape victims. The list should be prepared with the cooperation of refugee counsellors, relief workers and trained refugee interpreters to make sure that the suggested steps are culturally acceptable.

The role of religious leaders

Religious leaders can do a lot to help rape victims and to change negative attitudes towards them.

- Arrange meetings with religious leaders and community volunteers and helpers to discuss the problem of rape.

- Seek their help to stop negative attitudes towards victims and their families.

- Discuss the possibility of having special prayers and meetings for rape victims and their families. These meetings could be led by religious leaders in the community.

- Community leaders, including religious leaders (priests, mullahs, monks or other religious figures), must be made aware of their importance in the healing process of rape victims and their families. They can educate the men to be compassionate, and help change negative attitudes towards the victims.

Preventing the rape of refugee women

Relief workers, officials and representatives of nongovernmental organizations should together prepare guidelines for action when rape is reported in the camp. Host governments should also be included in planning the response. The guidelines should include a set of instructions for relief workers to follow when rape or sexual intimidation is reported. The procedure should be made known to the refugee women and their communities. They should know whom to consult when rape occurs. This is in itself a preventive measure against rape.

Service providers and mental health counsellors can do a lot through public education and advocacy to draw attention to, and deal with, the root causes of rape. Because refugees themselves do not hold positions of authority, they rely on higher authorities for assistance. Sharing information with policy-makers and decision-makers will enable them to help prevent rape becoming a continuing problem in the refugee community.

Some guidelines for collecting information on rape

1. Keep records on the number of refugee women and girls who have been raped. Also record the number of rapes occurring each week or each month and each year.

2. Make sure that information is general and does not in any way identify the victims.

3. Call together a "protection group" of professionals, service providers and camp authorities to meet regularly to plan and manage a systematic way of protecting against rape in the refugee community.

4. Encourage higher authorities to prepare articles on rape and sexual violence for newspapers and other communications media, and to prepare information for human rights reports.

5. Try to arrange for officials of the host country to be included in the protection group and to report their activities in assisting rape victims. Ask that representatives of international agencies follow up their agreements with host countries and other authorities in writing.

6. Tell others success stories about rape victims who have overcome their problems.

7. Do not house rape victims separately. This will draw negative attention to them in the community.

The organization of services that promote the mental health and well-being of refugees

This manual is primarily for workers in camps for refugees or other displaced persons. It aims to help them to deal with the mental health problems of persons who have fled their homes and, in many cases, their countries also. It does not deal in detail with broader issues, largely because it was felt that the potential readers would not be in a position to take decisions affecting the running of the camp as a whole. However, it may be worth while to give here a few suggestions about how life in a refugee camp might be organized to take account of people's mental as well as physical needs. These ideas are mentioned with only brief notes rather than detailed suggestions about how they could be implemented. In part, this is because methods of implementation have to be geared to specific situations in refugee camps, to structures that are already set up and to the predominant culture of those living there. For this reason, mechanisms have to be found to encourage the refugees or other displaced persons themselves, as far as possible, to take charge of those aspects of camp life that affect their mental well-being. If refugees are to take charge, this means they should have a powerful say in what is done. It may mean leaving some things completely in the hands of people from within the refugee community.

The point of this is not just to ensure that what is done is culturally appropriate. Obtaining broad participation and giving a say to the refugees or other displaced persons prevents the harmful sense of helplessness and enforced dependence which can drain their energy. The refugees themselves, if encouraged, will bring up their own ideas of things that can be done, and although these may seem difficult to accomplish they should be considered and possibly tried. In a situation of demoralization, lack of resources and lack of access to things that used to be a normal part of life, some refugees may become violent and commit criminal acts, taking advantage of weaker and more vulnerable people in the camp. By encouraging mutual support groups and possibly providing the means for them to meet, morale can be raised and measures put in place whereby people can protect each other. If people see that they have some power to control their lives and environment, they can be encouraged to improve both their camp environment and their health. This can produce a circle of benefit whereby as refugees see that they can actually improve things, their feeling of power grows and they feel encouraged to take on more challenges.

The provision of employment is of course very difficult in camps for refugees or displaced persons, and usually only very few persons will be able to get work. However, the provision of tools and materials for cultivating or building can allow people to do things for themselves. Refugees and other displaced persons can be encouraged to organize their own leisure-time activities, and again a small amount of resources may be provided to make it possible for culturally appropriate activities to take place.

Although it may be administratively easier to divide up families, providing one set of accommodation for men and another for women with their children, every effort should be made to avoid doing this. Some way of allowing families a little privacy, if only by hanging clothes or mats between the spaces allocated to them, may also help. In all these matters, of course, the refugees' own wishes, customs and suggestions need to be taken into account. Although families should be kept together, thought should be given to allow for the organization of crèches and day care for children. This can possibly be done using a rota system whereby parents share the reponsibility of care, taking turns in looking after a group of children. This allows parents to have time to do things away from their children.

During the first influx of a large number of refugees or displaced persons, the physical demands for food and shelter are greatest. It is tempting for assisting agencies to continue to be preoccupied with these matters, forgetting that once these needs have been attended to — even partially — mental health needs are of equal importance. The raising and maintaining of the morale of the refugees and other displaced persons become concerns that should never be ignored. A small investment in this area will pay enormous dividends, not just for mental health but for physical health as well.